OWN IT

THE SMART ORTHODONTIST'S GUIDE TO

THE SMART ORTHODONTIST'S GUIDE TO

STANDING OUT IN A CROWDED MARKET

D1081657

DUSTIN S. BURLESON, DDS, MBA

Copyright © 2018 by Dr. Dustin S. Burleson, MBA.

All rights reserved. No part of this book may be used or reproduced in any manner whatsoever without prior written consent of the author, except as provided by the United States of America copyright law.

Published by Advantage, Charleston, South Carolina.
Member of Advantage Media Group.

ADVANTAGE is a registered trademark, and the Advantage colophon is a trademark of Advantage Media Group, Inc.

Printed in the United States of America.

10 9 8 7 6 5 4 3 2 1

ISBN: 0991346874
LCCN: 2011000000

Cover design by Art in Motion Graphic Design LLC
Layout design by Art in Motion Graphic Design LLC

This publication is designed to provide accurate and authoritative information in regard to the subject matter covered. It is sold with the understanding that the publisher is not engaged in rendering legal, accounting, or other professional services. If legal advice or other expert assistance is required, the services of a competent professional person should be sought.

Advantage Media Group is proud to be a part of the Tree Neutral® program. Tree Neutral offsets the number of trees consumed in the production and printing of this book by taking proactive steps such as planting trees in direct proportion to the number of trees used to print books. To learn more about Tree Neutral, please visit **www.treeneutral.com**.

Advantage Media Group is a publisher of business, self-improvement, and professional development books and online learning. We help entrepreneurs, business leaders, and professionals share their Stories, Passion, and Knowledge to help others Learn & Grow. Do you have a manuscript or book idea that you would like us to consider for publishing? Please visit **advantagefamily.com** or call **1.866.775.1696**.

TABLE OF CONTENTS

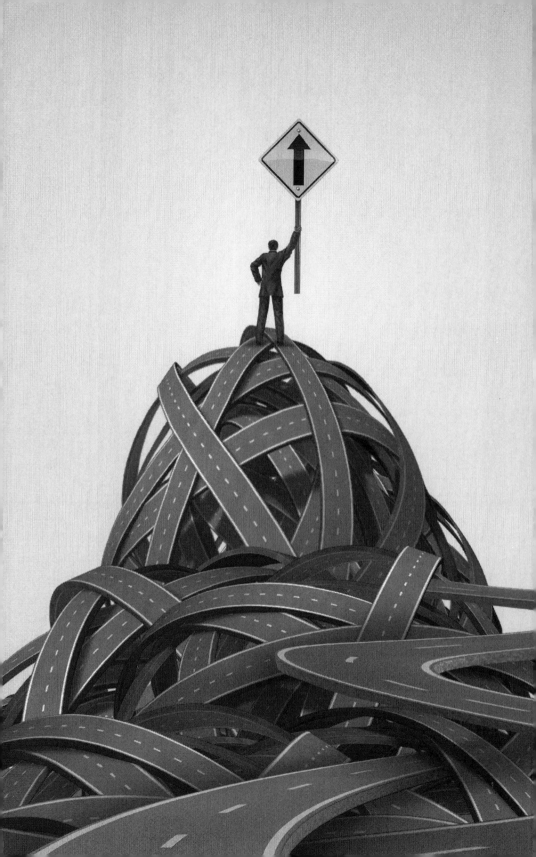

CHAPTER ONE
INTRODUCTION

"Stay hungry, stay foolish." – Steve Jobs

If you are picking up this book, there is a darn good chance you already know what it is that you want to do in life. Chances are, you are an orthodontist or are interested in becoming one. Most people have already defined what it is that they want to do, such as become the "best orthodontist" in a particular area. Yet less than 5% of those people will actually own that position. That's a big mistake, and one that will cost you and your practice dearly if it's not turned around.

It's one thing to say you want to be the best, but truly owning it is something all together different. Owning it means that you stand behind your work and you provide a satisfaction guarantee. Period. If people are not happy with you, then they get their money back, no questions asked. That's owning it. That takes guts and an amount of grit that most people just simply don't have. But it doesn't stop there.

Owning it also means that you do the unnecessary. You remember your patients' names, you send them gifts, you do things to wow the people and keep them talking. You go above and beyond, without it feeling like you are having to go above and beyond, because it's just who you are and what you do. It's a part of you and your practice.

By owning it, you also do something that is rarely ever heard of in business, let alone the orthodontic field – you admit when you are wrong and you apologize for it. We can all agree that humans are imperfect and you are going to make mistakes. Granted, it has to be a small percentage of them if you want your doors to stay open, but they are going to happen from time to time. When they happen, you don't hide behind policy or blame others. If the patient has

1

decalcification, for example, you can either blame the patient or you can blame your inability to properly motivate people to take the braces off a long time ago. You have to own it and then do whatever it takes to fix it.

I can share with you my own experience in owning it and taking responsibility. I've paid for veneers and composites in too many patients to count, and in turn, those patients are raving fans of mine. They send me ten times more referrals than the cosmetic dentistry cost me. Plus, referring doctors see how committed you are to excellence. Trust me when I say that you will likely be the only orthodontist in your area who behaves like this, which is exactly what you want.

Anyone can say that their business is exceptional, but only doctors who own it can actually show you the proof.

Many people don't know what it means to own it, nor do they know how to make it happen. They also don't know why it should matter to them and what it can do for their practice, which is why I wrote this book. There are a few major things that will happen when you own it, including:

- Your revenue and profit will be in the top 1-5% of the profession.
- Your employee productivity will grow beyond $400,000 in revenue per employee.

- Referrals will represent a majority of your new patients.
- New patient conversion will increase to 85% or higher.
- You will garner a lot of attention in the media.
- Your fees will tolerate much more elasticity, as you're paid for who you are, not what you do.

If these are things that all sound good to you, and they should sound fantastic, then owning it is certainly the right path for you to take. Before we go any further, though, it's important for me to disclose that owning it isn't for sissies. No, it's not for everyone and not everyone will be able to pull it off. Owning it takes dedication, hard work, and a commitment to the idea and principles of owning it. If you fall short, then so too will the benefits you would have received from owning it. If you stick with it, stay the course, and remain committed to owning it, then you will see the beautiful results. But it's not for everyone. It's only for those who want to go to the extra mile in order to be on top.

My Story

People often wonder who I am to share my story and dish out the advice that I do. Well, I will tell you that I grew up in the world of dentistry. I am one of 12 in my family, so you can imagine what family picture day looks like. Dads, brothers, uncles, cousins, ex-wife, her dad, and just about everyone in the family is a dentist. I remember when I was a child spending time in my dad's basement riding around on my Big Wheel, immersed in dentistry. When I was in the eighth grade I was doing his payroll, and by the time I was in high school I was running his office. I even computerized the entire practice.

The dental field is in my blood and it's what I know. I don't offer the advice I make based on outside observations. I'm right there in it with you all, in the trenches, seeing what works and what doesn't. I know these things from experience and from the years that I've spent researching the field and providing consulting services to many in the field around the world. I live it, I breathe it, and well, *I own it.*

Being that I sign payroll checks, too, I'm right there with you all. I'm an orthodontist and have been one since 2006. I'm actually right there with you, treating patients and signing paychecks. We built my practice from scratch and focused on doing some great things with our patients, so we treat a lot of difficult patients there. We do a lot of surgery cases, cleft palate, and even did NAM exclusively in the practice for years and took it to the hospital.

I know the challenges every orthodontic practice has in trying to build a patient base and striving to become the best in their area. In fact, our practice is in Kansas City, where there are two million people and 72 orthodontists. I love to joke about how 10 of us could drop dead and nobody would even know. I came into a market that already had plenty of orthodontists, so I decided that owning it was going to be the best route of attack to get my fair share of the market. I started to look for ways to treat patients who were probably going to have a difficult time getting treatment otherwise. These included the people who other orthodontists turned away, because it required surgery, as well as people who felt they couldn't have treatment because of scheduling constraints and their finances.

For the first three years after hanging out our shingle, we straightened teeth, did a lot of cleft palate care, which other orthodontists don't do, and I was just your bread-and-butter orthodontist. I took care of a lot of hairy cases and we grew it to where I thought we were doing pretty well. The problem was that we had created a system that was extremely stressful to everyone involved, including me and the entire team. I knew that something had to change. Either we needed to sell the practice, file bankruptcy, or walk away from it. In fact, on a cold day in February 2009, my entire team walked out, and I went to lunch to ponder my options and find the silver lining.

We built a practice that was perfect for the patients. They loved our office. But we had totally forgotten about the employees. In addition to my staff walking out on me all at once, I've had embezzlement issues three times, I've survived board complaints from jealous competitors and I've survived more audits and lawsuits than most doctors face in ten lifetimes.

I've made every mistake there is to make. I've done every dumb thing there is to do, but I've learned from every one of them, and I've used that information to further our growth and strengthen our mission and purpose. Today, we have multiple locations and doctors, we've added a pediatric dentistry and now treat over 11,000 active patients. In our largest clinic, we operate 22 chairs from 7am-7pm, six days per week.

In this book and elsewhere, I don't share my embarrassing failures because I am proud of them. Trust me when I say they were each a huge pain that cost me time and money and made me question what the hell I was doing and thinking. In 2009, I had to figure it out, and fast, or I was not going to survive. Everything I learned and experienced to grow my practices dramatically and quickly I share with you, so that you can learn from them too. I would prefer they don't happen to you, but the honest truth is that some of these things, and many others, are going to happen to you. The secret is how you respond with confidence.

Everything is not perfect in my world, or yours, and I would never want someone to tell you that it is. There's not a lot you can learn when things are going well. No one ever became an experienced sailor on a calm, sunny day. There is plenty to learn, however, when the clouds roll in and the winds pick up. When the sea gets rough, real sailors are made. Perhaps this is why I'm much more interested in discussing my horrible outcomes with a colleague. What do we learn by talking about our best cases? Everyone knows what a perfect occlusion looks like. It's the case with 28 broken brackets, white spots and wicked gingival overgrowth that we can learn something from.

The Approach

My approach to what we've done in our practice and what I'm going to share with you is to help you see things through a little different lens. My wish is that we can learn from a lot of mistakes. Maybe we can learn from a lot of things that no one else will share with you. When I started sharing my stories and experiences, other orthodontists started seeking us out and wanting to come see our practice. They would fly to Kansas City, sit in one of our offices, and they would observe and ask questions. We'd pick each other's brains, more or less, and then they would head back home filled with lots of new information and ideas. Even when we started charging for the coaching services, they still kept flying in for the experience and insight that they could take back to their own practice.

Let me divulge how I have also learned a great deal about how practices are run and what makes for good and bad practice. We conduct a "secret shopper" service, where we send in actual patients for treatment at orthodontic practices around the country. In fact, I have more secret shopper data from actual orthodontic patients than any other person on the planet. I have lots of data about actual patients in the wild. If you were to study animals, you would go to the zoo or jungle. I wanted to study patients and the process, so I went to orthodontic practices around the country.

I've studied patients, over 10,000 hours of secret shopper video, and I've read the patient-completed assessments, and the assessments completed by the treatment coordinators and doctors. We have tons and tons of data. What we have learned is something that can seriously change your life if you pay attention. We have learned things about how to better greet the patient, about our uniforms, what we did in the first four minutes of the patient exam, and more. We took that information and used it to make changes in our practice and our conversion rate went from 50% to 85%, just with those minor changes throughout the course of what we were doing. **What would an increase of 30% more in new patients do for *your* business?**

Game Changing

Through all of my consultation, research, and my own experiences, I have come up with information that will be life-changing for you and your practice. I've broken it down into what I feel are the 15 most important core areas that I see missing in almost every one of the secret shopper tapes. *These are the 15 things that every orthodontist must address in order to grow their practice and really thrive.* I also think that at least 95% of the orthodontist practices out there can make improvements in these 15 core areas.

My goal is not to make you feel that you have to exactly replicate everything I'm doing in my practice or to say that the way I'm showing you is the only way it should be done. Maybe you don't like some of the things that I will propose, have reasons for doing it another way, or maybe the big goals for your practice are not the same as they are for mine. For whatever the reason, it's fine. It is not my goal to say this is the only way. My goal in sharing this information that I've spent years gathering is to help you learn how to think about it accurately. If you were to watch 10,000 hours of patient videos over my shoulder, your jaw would hit the floor at some of the things you would see. I should mention that we even secret shop our own offices every month at a minimum, so that we can spot something that's not right immediately, before it begins to drag our conversion rate down. I don't want anything loose to fall through the cracks. If our conversion rate slips, I will send in even more mystery shoppers, so we can spot exactly what the problem is and get it corrected right away.

My favorite quote is, "There are no shortcuts to anywhere worth going." I live that with my practice. If you want to grow your practice, there are no easy buttons to push. *My goal is to help you own what you sell.* Just like when you think about companies like Uber or Domino's Pizza. You may think that Uber sells rides, but they don't. They are not selling transportation, they are selling time and convenience. They have defined it and own it.

When you think about Domino's Pizza, your first thought that comes to mind might be that they sell pizza. Come on, have you tried their "pizza" and really tasted it? It's a lot like cardboard with ketchup on it. Selling pizza is not what they have owned. They are in the business of pizza delivery. If you want a great-tasting, authentic pizza, you probably have a great little Italian restaurant you will go pick your pizza up from, or take the family there to dine out. But

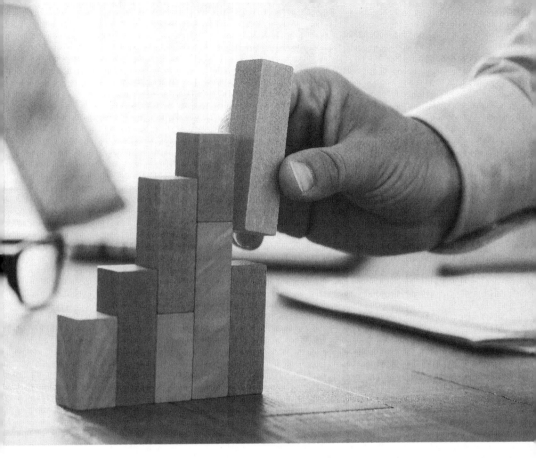

when you want pizza delivered, to save you time and make it more convenient, then you think of Domino's. Their mission is to deliver hot pizza to your door quickly. They don't promise that it's the best tasting pizza around, they just promise that it will be there fast.

Think about Apple for a moment, and most people would say that they sell computers, hardware, and phones. But that's not what they sell anymore. Apple is now a software business and they are really in the app business. Their products are just modes to deliver their software. They are really in the media and entertainment business and now even selling finance through Apple Pay. What it looks like on the surface that they are selling, the devices, is not at all what they are selling. Those devices are tools to make it possible to sell you what they are really in the business of selling.

All three of these companies, Uber, Domino's Pizza, and Apple, have defined what it is that they do well, and they own it. They excel at it and they continue to see growth in their annual earnings. In a time when people are hurried, busy, and distracted, these companies have owned what they do well, and have flourished as a result.

How do these stories correlate with your practice? Well, what do most orthodontists think they sell? Braces, or straight teeth, maybe confidence, or try inserting any phrase here. But what are you really selling? Well, yes, you are selling braces, Invisalign, straight teeth, better occlusion, health, beauty, and whatever else. But the 10,000 hours of secret shopper data that I have far and above disputes and throws into massive disarray the assumption that you sell braces. When you think you sell braces and focus on that, your conversion rate is and will always be around 50% of your new patients. When you think about this differently, you see growth like Domino's, you see growth like Uber, and you will see growth like Apple.

I know you may be feeling right now like your head is going to explode, because you believe you are in the business of selling braces. But you are not in the business of selling braces. You are in the human capital business, you're in the logistics business, you're in the communications business, you're in the marketing business, in sales, and in networking. You are also in the psychology business, the hospitality business, and also in the live events business. You are in the public relations and media business, in the education business, and the transportation business if you have multiple locations or you deliver retainers to patients like we often do. You are also in the real estate business if you own your practices, or even if you don't, because you are kind of playing in that world. You are also in the philanthropy business and the innovation business. You can see where I'm going with this.

Now, before you freak out, throw the book down, and say you can't possibly wear that many hats, just bear with me here. The great thing is that you don't have to pick all of them to own. You just need to pick one. It doesn't matter which one it is, but you have to pick one and own it. Do it better than it has ever been done before. Maybe you decide to focus on owning how you hire and train employees. It doesn't matter which one you want to focus on, but you have to pick one, own it, and then do it better than anyone else ever has.

This is a great exercise in creative thinking and in stimulating your practice. Once you pick which one you are going to own, then you need to put a moat around it. Tell the world that you own it and you do it better than anyone else has before. Right now, you don't know which one of these things you want to pick and own, and that's OK. That is what this book is about. I am going to share with you the 15 core areas that I've narrowed down from my research. You can learn about each one and then make the decision which one you want to own. The one you own will most likely jump out at you, because it's going to be one that you see yourself in when you read it. It's something that you probably already love doing and you can see yourself owning it and doing it better than anyone else.

In the following chapters, you will learn about each of the 15 core areas and what you can do to own it, if you choose to. You may be skeptical about some of the areas and others will make perfect sense to you, leaving you to wonder how you never thought about it before. My hope is that you finish this book with a new outlook on each of these 15 core areas. They are not the things you were taught in college and you will not hear them from anyone else in the business. I'm sharing them with you, because I know how much they matter, and I know how much picking one of them and owning it matters.

No, you are not in the business of selling braces. If that's what you have been thinking all these years, or for as long as you have been in the field, then I'm hopefully about to change that mentality. When you have a better understanding of what it is that you are really selling, then the sky is the limit.

When you pick something and own it, doing it better than anyone else, you will see your practice grow like never before. I may hold the record on the amount of orthodontic secret shopper data, but it would never be worth much if I didn't share it with every orthodontist in the world, so that they can use it to grow their practices and we can use it to move our profession in the right direction.

"The path to success is to take massive, determined action." - Tony Robbins

---

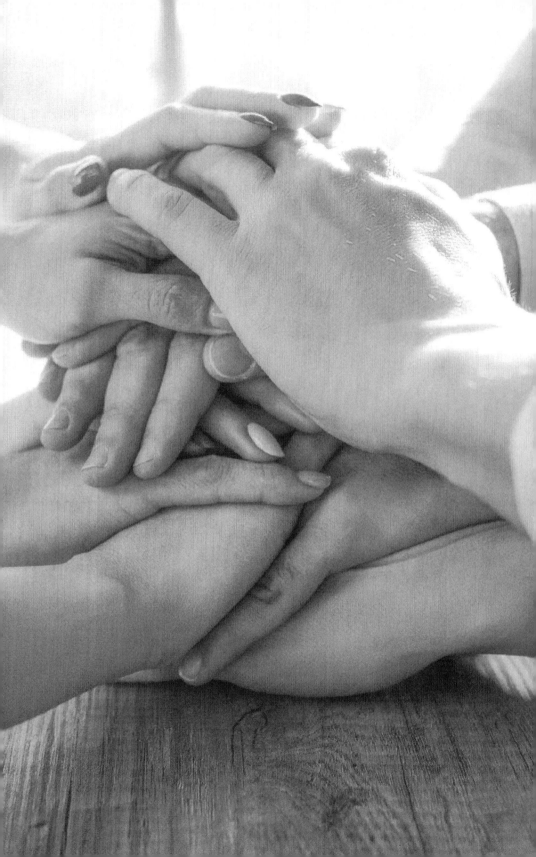

CHAPTER TWO
HUMAN CAPITAL

"Start with good people, lay out the rules, communicate with your employees, motivate them and reward them. If you do all those things effectively, you can't miss."
- Lee Iacocca

As clear cut as what Lee Iacocca says about taking care of employees is, most of the time it falls on deaf ears. It sure did for me, and I know it does for the many orthodontists who I have consulted and watched secret shopper videos on. *Human capital is one of our greatest assets,* but more often than not, we fail to remember that in the process, we fail our practice and the patients.

I've shared my story before about how I went to lunch one cold winter day and came back to my entire staff walking out on me. I don't mean they handed in a two-week notice or said they were taking off the rest of the afternoon. I mean they collectively were sick of the bullshit and had decided together that they would walk out, leaving me to see 38 patients that afternoon all on my own. That was a wake-up call like you could not imagine.

When you everyone in your office quits at the same time, you know there's something drastically wrong. The writing was on the wall all along, but I was so caught up in my own thoughts that I couldn't see past them to realize I had an unhappy team. They were more than unhappy. They were at the point where they figuratively said "screw you," and they all walked out, leaving my jaw to hit the ground, and my ego to have to take a back seat. It was time for me to realize that maybe I *didn't* have all my ducks in a row and that there were things I should be doing better. A *lot* better.

Human capital is one of the 15 core areas that will make or break your practice, just as it did mine. You don't want to wait until the point when your staff all walk out on you for the message to hit you over the head. *Knowing that human capital in your practice is extremely important is where it starts.* Knowing how to cultivate that to your benefit is where you want to be, and I'll show you how to get there.

Hiring Right, Setting the Stage

If you are like just about all other orthodontists, you are not all that into the act of hiring and training your employees. I get it, I was there as well. It's something you know needs to be done, but you don't really like the stuff, so maybe you hire an office manager to do the job. Maybe your office manager digs the hiring process, but isn't all that keen on supervising and making sure that people are actually doing what they are supposed to be doing, and calling them on it when they are not.

One of the important things to remember here is that it's not an "us and them" mentality. It's not that there is you and then there is your staff. Your staff are part of the entire show in your office. Walt Disney set the lead on this issue, when he said that those who worked in Disneyland and Disney World were not employees, but they were cast members. He considered his theme parks a show, and every employee, or cast member, was part of the show. It's no different with your own team. They are not something that is an outside entity or added-on piece. They are part of the show in your practice. Every person on your team is playing a role in the show.

If you were to take an objective look at your office and be honest about it, how does it make you feel? How do you view it? What would I think if I walked in tomorrow and took a look around? Would I be able to see the drinks and snacks that employees have out in view of patients? What about papers on the floor, chipped paint on the walls, or a dirty coffee machine? Would there be cobwebs in the corners? Take a good look around your office when your team is there doing what they do and take a mental note of all of these things. See it as if you are seeing it for the first time, so you notice what others see when they walk into your office.

Now, how would your office look if you knew that tomorrow the president was going to be stopping in? My guess is that you would spend some time cleaning it up. The beverages would be hidden, the papers picked up, the chipped paint repaired, and even that ripped chair would be fixed or replaced. All of this, how your office looks, is also part of the show. It's the stage and you need your stage to look and feel the part. It needs to be kept to look like you are expecting the president to arrive at any minute. When you visit Disney World, it's not just the buildings and the rides that are kept in good order for their guests. It's everything on the property. From the parking lot to the restrooms to the walkways and benches that you can sit and rest on, everything is well maintained and kept as if the president may arrive that day.

Think about the last production show you attended. If you have ever been to Broadway, then you know a show like the Nutcracker is filled with highly talented people. The team that will put that show on is part of the show and they never once forget their role. Sure, they have problems just like everyone else, but when they step on that stage nothing else matters. You know things are going on their lives, just like everyone else's, but to watch them perform you wouldn't know it. Whether they just broke up with their boyfriend, were evicted from their apartment, recently lost their grandmother, or their child was just diagnosed with cancer, they don't let it show. Their focus is to put on an amazing show for the audience, each and every time.

They do that because of the expectations that have been set. How you hire, interview, train, supervise, and motivate your people has everything to do with how you see their role in your show.

Employees Matter

What your employees bring to the show is far greater than what you have likely been suspecting all along. You know they are there, doing their tasks and contributing, but you have likely thought of them as an add-on, rather than a part of it all. When we can change that, we will provide a better experience for our patients, as well as make our office a pleasant place to work. Your employees know whether or not you truly value them and their contribution, despite or even with what you may say to them. They feel it in the core of their being, and how you make them feel about their role in the show will have a huge difference in how they perform.

Disney is a man I greatly admire and a company that my family loves. I've learned a lot of great business advice from Disney, including that you never know where your next big idea is going to come from. Several times per year, we take our people to the Disney Institute because they have some really cool things they do that most other companies don't do. We've even brought them to Kansas City to spend time with our coaching clients.

Phil Holmes, who is the vice president at Magic Kingdom, inside one of the Disney parks, oversees some 70,000 employees. The park itself has 40 square miles, which is the size of many cities, and it's the largest site employer in the United States. You would think that he'd be untouchable to those employees, but that's not the case at all. They actually publish his voicemail to make it accessible for all cast members. Any employee, even on their first day on the job, whether they are pushing the hot dog cart, sweeping the floors, cleaning the restrooms, or running rides, has the ability to leave a voicemail for the VP. Why does he do that? Because Walt was right, when he said that you never know where your best idea is going to come from. It could come from one of your employees. Without them having access to share it, that idea may never be heard.

We watch our secret shopper videos, we evaluate the treatment coordinators doing their assessment, then the doctors doing their own assessment, and we talk about what it is that they see. It may surprise you to learn that the best ideas come from the treatment coordinator and from the front desk, rather than from the doctor. It's just the opposite of what you would think, but they see things from a different perspective, which gives them some insight that you may not have.

Disney has a "You Ask, We Listen" philosophy, and every one of those voicemails they get are listened to. They even post responses to them in the employee newsletter that goes out to every employee. We stole the You Ask, We Listen idea right from them and we put it on our newsletter, which we send out via direct mail, even though I know they could go download it online and get it sent to their email. I want to make sure they see their ideas are considered, shared, and things are followed through. I want them to know just how damn important I think their ideas are and that when they think they

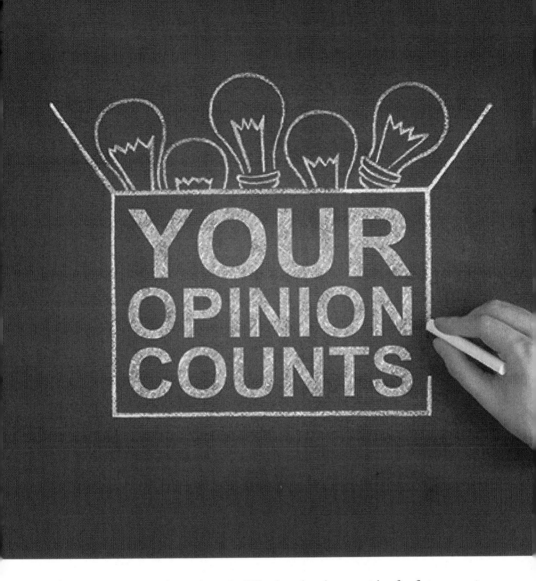

have one, I want to hear about it. Whether they have an idea for fixing a major problem in how we deliver retainers or how we get Invisalign trays back, or how we ship out things to other offices, I'm all ears.

Howard Schultz, of Starbucks fame, has an effective philosophy when it comes to listening to employees. He believes that if you are the janitor, then you should be the one picking out the broom. What does the office manager know about picking out the broom? The guy sweeping the floors knows what is going to work best and should be the one picking it out. Listen to their ideas and things will become more effective and productive. All the same, what do I know about distal end cutters? I honestly don't have a clue, but guess who does? The clinic assistants do. One day, our clinical assistant told me that we needed some better distal end cutters, because we were shipping them out every 10 seconds to get them repaired, because we see so many patients. I asked her if she'd like to do some homework to research which ones are the best, get some samples, and bring in some people to see which ones are the best. "Yeah, I'd love to do that," she said. And that's how things get done. When you listen for good ideas, your employees will bring them to you.

Another idea that we got from Disney to elicit feedback and ideas from our team members is to put a huge dry erase board up in the break room. You can get them at an office supply store or print shop. Listen to your team members, and when they let you know what's not working right, put it on the board and date it. Whether it's a complaint about parking, health benefits, the retirement program, or the kind of toilet paper being used in the restroom. Whatever it is that is frustrating them needs to go on that board so they know you are working on it. I keep it on that board to let them know that I'm aware of the situation and that it's being worked on. The idea is that next month they will hopefully see a checkmark next to it, so that they know the source of frustration has been rectified, or there's a notation to let them know that progress has been made.

Employee Engagement

Since the late 1990s, Gallup has been tracking employee engagement. This gives us some insight as to how engaged or connected employees feel to their job and place of employment. There's no doubt that you have dealt with numerous businesses in the past where you could tell the employee was not at all engaged. They could have been watching paint dry just the same as they were doing their job. We've all observed this, but we don't always realize the impact it can have on our practice, or why this happens. The more we understand it, the more we can use that information to make changes for the better in our own practice and with our employees.

For the last few years, Gallup has reported that employee engagement is right around 32%. This means that only 32% of people are engaged in their job.

They also show that nearly 51% are not engaged at all, and another 17% are actively disengaged. If these numbers represent what's going on in your practice, as they do in the general workforce, it's a recipe for disaster. It's alarming, and if something isn't done to correct it your practice will suffer as a result, or will never reach the level of success that you have your heart set on. **You need engaged employees in order to become highly successful.**

To determine if employees are engaged, Gallup uses three key workplace elements, which include being able to do what each person does best on a daily basis, working with someone who encourages them to develop, and the person believing their opinion counts at work. In other words, those employees who are doing a job they are not trained for or are unsure of, and not working with someone who values their opinion, creates a situation where they will no longer be engaged. When employees are not engaged, your office will suffer.

Gallup has advised that *"Engaged employees support the innovation, growth and revenue that their companies need."* That's important information that every orthodontist should take notice of. If you want your practice to be innovative, grow, and reach your revenue goals you will need to have employees who are engaged or it's just not likely to happen.

So how the heck do you go about engaging your employees? There are plenty of things you can do, starting with the ones I've already mentioned. When you make your employee suggestions something that you want, something that you listen to and value, and take action on, then you will engage them. They will know you care about how they feel about their place of employment. Your team members see things that you can't see when it comes to the practice and patient experience. Let them express that, use the information to make improvements, and they will become engaged. In fact, when your employees know you value their ideas and input, they will do everything they can to help you reach your goals.

You can improve engagement by making it a part of your human capital strategy. This includes having good leadership, communication systems, clarifying what the work expectations are, ensuring employees receive proper training and development tools, instilling a positive atmosphere in the office and among all team members, and giving people the opportunity to use their strengths at work. Doing these things doesn't take a huge effort on your part, but it does take a commitment to human capital. When you are committed to your employees and want them to love their experience working for you, they will in turn be fully engaged and committed to you and your practice. The only way your practice can become highly successful is for that to happen. My practice could not be what it is today if only one out of every three people in the office was engaged. Your practice can never become as successful as you'd like it to be if over half of your employees are not at all engaged in what they are doing for the show.

Owning It

If you remember, I said you don't need to own every one of the 15 core areas that are laid out in this book. You can pick just one of them and own it. If you are going to own human capital, then you are going to make the decision that you will have the best damn orthodontic practice to work for in the entire area. I don't mean that you will just be average or slightly above average. I mean that employees will talk and word will get around that your practice is amazing to work for, that you care about your employees, what they think, they want, and you give them the opportunity to show their skills, contribute, and to strengthen the company. When you do that, you will create an unstoppable force that will help propel your practice to the top.

In order for any business to accomplish anything at all, it must rely upon human capital. It's a magnificent resource that has been taken for granted for far too long. Your office should never be a revolving door for employees. If it is, that's a huge red flag that there's a problem and you need to address it right away. Owning human capital means that you are going to be committed to hiring the right people for every position, ensuring that people receive the training and development tools they need at every juncture, empowering them, and letting them know their opinions are valued. There are many ways to do that, including things like the employee newsletter, the white board in the break room, and the VP of Disney having a voicemail that every employee has access to.

If you were to add up the salary of every employee you have, you would see a rough image of what it costs you every year. But that's only half the picture. That shows you all of your out-of-pocket expenses of having your team, but it doesn't show you the revenue you are leaving behind by ensuring they are engaged on the job. If you could see the dollar amount of what you are leaving behind by having employees who are not engaged, you would probably be blown away. It's costing you new patients, referrals, conversions, and so much more. It's even costing you more time being spent at home with your family and being able to really enjoy your vacation when you take one, rather than having to constantly keep tabs on what is going in the office because you don't fully trust leaving them on their own.

Human capital is your practice's greatest asset, but if you are like most orthodontists you have likely been drastically overlooking it for years. Deciding to own it is a decision that will completely change your practice. It's going to start with you, as you begin to see your employees differently, and then it's going to resonate throughout the whole office. You will be amazed at what happens when you own it, tap into it, and let the magic happen and you begin to see the results that come.

Everyone on the planet wants to be recognized and valued. When I see that the top 5% of orthodontists have one of the 15 core areas owned, I know that they have the happiest patients around. They are the ones doing the coolest things with their kids and their spouses, they are giving the most to charity, and they are growing the highest net incomes. These 15 core areas, human capital included, are the stones you want to turn over and look under. I've watched too many new patients come into too many offices where it is clear and obvious that no one's focusing on how the office has hired, trained, supervised, and motivated their employees. For too many people it's clearly just a job. No one is playing a role in the show.

Owning it means that you want your employees to play a role in the show, and believe me when I say that it will make a world of difference for both them and your practice.

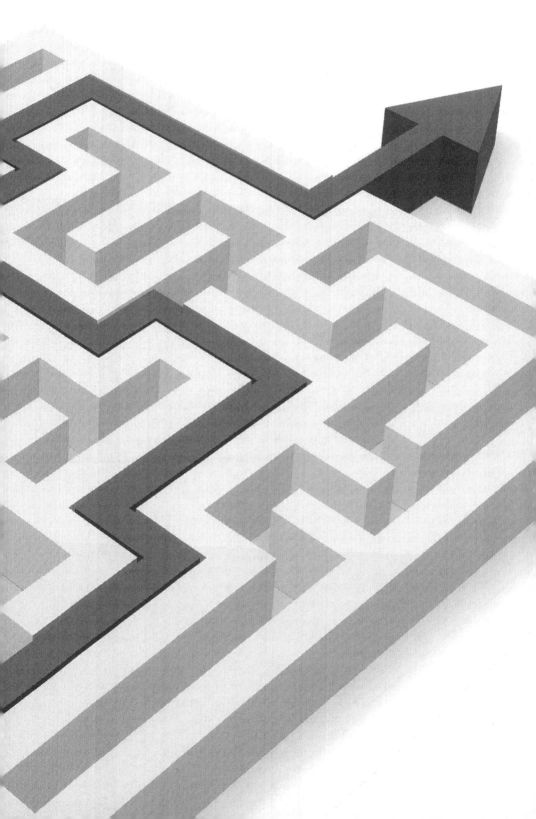

CHAPTER THREE
LOGISTICS

"It's okay to have your eggs in one basket as long as you control what happens to that basket." – Elon Musk

The second of the 15 core areas that you should consider owning is logistics. It's not an area that most people own, but doing so would bring about many benefits for your practice. Over the years I've come to see that there are certain orthodontists who have the ability to really own this area and should, because the nature of what it entails is just part of who they are and what they love to do.

Maybe you're a tech guy or the engineer type. Maybe you are someone who loves the spreadsheets and logistics that are involved in running your practice. Perhaps it's the inventory system that catches your eye and piques your interest, because you know full well it could be so much better than it is. Or it could be that your lab prescriptions and appliances cover the area that interests you. Maybe you get excited about the idea of drastically improving how they are made and delivered.

Defining Logistics
Logistics, by definition, is the handling of all of the details of an operation. In other words, it's how all of the details are handled at your practice. These include such things as coordination and supply chain management. It's not something that most people give much thought to, but it's something that has an incredible amount of power over how your practice is working. *The logistics of your office are something that will help make or break you, or if not break you, it can at the least hold you back from reaching your potential.* Poor logistics are like a bum leg. You may be able to keep moving forward, but you

will do so at a slower pace, and possibly even stumble some here and there as you make your way.

Owning the logistics in your practice helps ensure that you have what you need, when you need it, and things can keep moving along at a good pace. Good logistics help to improve efficiency, while poor logistics do the opposite. In your practice, your logistics are going to keep such things well oiled, such as inventory management, order fulfillment, scheduling, and coordinating.

When you take the time to own the logistics at your practice, you will be taking measures to improve everything from efficiency to productivity. By having systems in place and being organized, you are going to better serve your patients, save money, increase productivity, and increase your profits. Those are a lot of good reasons to consider your logistics and what you can do to make some improvements in this area.

When you keep up with inventory and placing the orders for what you need and when you will need it, there is a good chance you will save money. The items will be there when your team members need them, and you may get discounts from ordering on time, in bulk, and not needing last minute rush orders to be delivered that you may be stuck paying a premium for. Your productivity increases because there are no slowdowns and nothing is held back. Your staff can do their jobs, keeping the flow going, rather than stopping at random times because things are out of stock, not organized, or they don't know the appropriate procedures to follow.

Being able to increase profitability is always a nice draw, and nailing down your logistics is a way to help you do just that. *By becoming more efficient, your team will be more productive, and more productivity equals more profitability.* You want your practice to run like a well-oiled machine, and the only possible way you can do that is to take on your logistics and manage them better than you have ever dreamed they could be done.

There's another benefit of having an office that is running more efficiently, too. You will have less stress and your work environment will be more enjoyable. When people can do their work and keep plugging along without getting tripped up over details, such as procedures not being followed or the stock

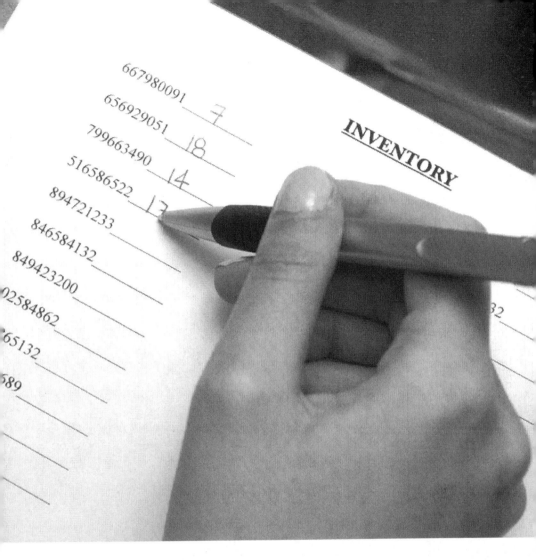

of necessary items being depleted, they will find their work experience more pleasing. Less stress is always a good thing for you and for everyone on your team. Your patients will find it more enjoyable, as well. They can tell when your staff is stressed, because they can feel it in their energy. When things go smoother for you and your team, they will also go smoother for your patients.

Our Logistics Experience

Whether you are excited by making improvements in the ordering systems or keeping inventory well stocked, logistics may be the area for you to own. In our practice, we sell a lot of whitening and it is shipped directly to the patient.

This is an area that one can own and excel in starting with the inventory control, how the orders are fulfilled, and who's in charge of the process. Not owning this area can lead to problems. We had issues with our inventory, so we went back and re-evaluated our process. We knew we were tired of not having the things on hand when we needed them, so we read a lot of information on the topic and created a new visual system. If you have seen our lab in the clinic you can see our visual inventory system. No one has to go searching through a storage closet for materials or supplies. A visual inventory, which we learned from the Toyota Motor Company, allows our employees to glance and see if we're out of any instruments, materials or supplies. We don't have to go hunting them down to investigate the state of our inventory or if we are getting low.

I don't need scanners, barcodes, and "advanced" inventory systems. We like to keep things simple and manageable. We've broken it down by location in the business. So you can actually sit and stare at what needs to be ordered in the coffee bar area and quickly know if we have enough on hand or not. This is something we do on a weekly basis. Every week, every office and with everything we order down to the paper clips, copier paper and creamer for the coffee. Everything is on a list and stored in a visual inventory system so it can be quickly replaced the minute a supervisor approves the order.

Maybe streamlining your logistics is something you need to improve. Look for every repetitive movement and potential bottleneck to delivering better service. When we did, we dramatically improved the efficiency of our lab scripts. We digitized them all and put them into our electronic patient record, so that every patient has every lab script filled out automatically just the way my system dictates. It makes it darn near impossible to screw up. We found a repetitive process and a bottleneck that was holding up appliance delivery for our patients. Automating and streamlining the process allows us to deliver appliances faster than our competitors and more accurately across multiple locations. We track them from start to finish, so that anyone in our organization can quickly and easily locate any appliance at any point in our supply chain. Patients and parents love the accuracy and convenience. They can have a scan or impression in one office location close to work and pick it up at an office location closer to home. Our focus on logistics has provided a competitive advantage in extreme patient convenience.

You may be at a point where you don't even know what kind of condition your logistics management is in. Many people don't, which is something I've learned through my consulting and our secret shopper videos. On the other hand, you may be someone who has been on top of it, kind of owning it all along, so you have a finger on what's going on and how it's all going. Either way, there are some great reasons for owning this area of your practice.

Once I saw the importance of owning the logistics area of our practice and what it could do for efficiency and productivity, there was no turning back. I can't imagine now going back to a time when we were not well organized, didn't have great procedures in plan that everyone is aware of, and would run out of necessary items. We have nailed the area of logistics. Sure, there are areas we will still continue to identify that we need to hone, but for now we have it down.

You will never regret owning the logistics of your practice. There will never be a day when you wish your team weren't working so efficiently and that productivity wasn't up. You won't wish that your inventory were a mess, and so on. But you will have many days where you regret not having those things in place, because you will feel it and you will see it. You will feel the frustration that you and your staff have when there's not an effective procedure in place or when inventory runs out of something you need to keep the flow going that day.

Owning It

So how do you go about owning the logistics in your office and what steps do you take to get there? While it may seem like this is an area that could be difficult to tackle, it's not going to be the mountain you may see it as. Yes, you do have to do the initial work to get these things into place, but once they are there it's just a matter of keeping up with them. That's not difficult to do, especially with a well-trained team.

There are many things you can do in the area of logistics to own them and make them work for your office, so that you gain the many benefits. While I will share some of the ways here, you will find that there are many others beyond this that will work well for your team or office.

Here are some areas to get you started with:

Assess Outcomes. Take the time to consider all of the possible outcomes and then determine what you need to do to be ready for them. This goes for ensuring your procedures are in place to making sure that you have the tools and supplies you need when you need them. Do you have a plan for what happens if someone cancels an appointment? What if a patient walks in the door asking for assistance for a broken bracket? What happens if your receptionist calls in sick, do you have a plan for who will take over that position and how the day will still carry on in a smooth manner, without the patients feeling the pinch of the person being out that day? While you may not be able to identify every single outcome that could happen, there are some that will be more common than others. Have the procedure in place for how to deal with it so that everyone knows right then, and the office will carry on without missing a beat.

Determine the resources needed. Take a look at all of the resources that are needed to support all of the office's objectives and operations. These are the things that should always be readily available. If they are not, then there is going to be a drag in the production and efficiency as people try to deal with what is missing. The good news here is that you can employ the assistance of your team to determine everything that is needed. They know what they need in order to do their job better than anyone else, so ask them what it is that they need. What do they think the patients need when they are in the waiting room, in the exam area, and what may they need when they head home? What do they feel is something that needs improving in the area of logistics, and while you are at it, solicit their ideas on how they feel the improvements can be made. In every position your team members fill, there are resources that are needed, just as there are resources needed for helping every patient. Evaluating what they are and then ensuring all the pieces are there when they are needed will keep your office running smoothly. Within this area, you will want to make it a priority to own ensuring your inventory and supplies are always maintained.

Have a vision. Part of the logistics for your office is to know what you want and where you want to go. It's not enough to just open your doors and let the chips fall where they may. You have to have a vision of what you want your practice to run like, and the ideas to help make it happen. With having a vision, you want to define a strategic direction for your office and have clear ideas of what's required. If you don't have a vision for your practice, then it's hard to ever reach those goals. You need to have a clear idea of what is required in order to meet the vision goals you have.

Become a planner. If you have always been someone who just does everything off the cuff, then you will need to make some changes in order to own the area of logistics. Owning this area is going to require that you become more of a planner. You will need to look ahead at situations, anticipate outcomes, and plan for things that can and do happen. It's going to require that you become meticulous with everything from your scheduling and new patient welcome kits being sent out to making sure that your waiting room has fresh magazines and a steady supply of coffee to keep waiting parents comfortable.

Improve relationships. With ensuring that you have everything you need when you need it, you will also want to improve relationships with people like your vendors. By ensuring you have good relationships with them, you will have a better chance at getting the things you need, knowing what's new and improved, and being able to find the best rates. When you have a good relationship with them they will want to play a role in helping to keep your office prepared for every patient. They may be able to bring things to your attention that you wouldn't otherwise notice, or they can help keep you up on products in the industry.

Look for efficiency. Owning logistics means that you will be identifying the most efficient systems around. You will want that for your office to show that you have the most efficient and smoothly running practice in the area. Seek out those highly effective systems and the best options possible that can be used to increase your efficiency and help your team become more effective. Owning logistics means you can't stay idle, doing something just because that's the way it has always been done. Rather, you will want to ask yourself and your team if there is a better way, a more efficient way, and then determine what it is and implement it into your procedures. Efficiency is the name of the game in logistics and needs to be a higher priority. Opt for the software and tools for each job that will help make it efficient, as well as accurate. In today's world, you may find that efficiency often lies in making the best use of technology, and if you do that is great. Embrace it, implement it and insure your team members are well trained on how you see it. At other times, however, you may find that efficiency comes in the simple old fashioned ways that things can be done. We don't always need to overthink an issue in order to find the most efficient solution for it, just as we want a quick visual model for keeping track of our inventory. Owning it means that you will do whatever it is that works best for your practice, whether that is turning to technology to automate and digitize, or doing things in a simpler manner that makes sense to you and your staff.

 Involve others. When you own logistics, it's not something you have to do all on your own, so don't think that this is going to become a huge burden on your shoulders. You won't forgo seeing patients so you can work on inventory and procedure protocol. Not at all. You will want to get your employees involved. Determine your vision and your objectives, and then share it with them, so they can all help to own the position of logistics. Let them know how important it is to you and why you are choosing to up your game, so they can get on board and help with it. The team can become a force that ensures procedures are in place, they are met, and that everything runs smoothly and efficiently. They can help identify areas that need to be addressed and ways that things can be made more efficient. Remember from the prior chapter: Your employees are your human capital, and they are a major benefit in your office. You just have to trust them enough to allow them to help strengthen your procedures and protocols. They will want to do it, especially if they see you trust them and value their input and efforts.

 Embrace organization. Being well organized is something that frankly scares the hell out of many people. They envision neatly stacked files and books, everything clean and in its place, and they fear they will never measure up. But being organized has some major perks, and it's part of handling the logistics at your office. When things are organized there is no guessing as to where everything is and whether you have inventory on hand. There is no wondering how to handle procedures or the possible things that may arise. Being organized means that your office is ready for what the day will bring, you know how to handle it, and you can do so efficiently. Being organized saves you time and money, and shows people you are on top of your game. Owning logistics means embracing more organization, determining where it can be used in your office, and how to best implement it. Again, it comes back to the point that doing this will help increase efficiency and productivity.

Making it Yours

If you choose to own logistics, you will be ensuring that your practice runs like a well-oiled machine and nothing short of that. There are no shortcuts and not meeting expectations in one area or another, because it's the area that you have committed to being the best at. It means you will be able to take on the minor details that end up having a major impact on how your office runs, and you will give them a fair evaluation to ensure that they are handled in the best possible manner for your office.

Don't you love when you walk into an office or business and everything runs smoothly? You can feel the energy in the air that they just know what they are doing, they are well prepared for you, and that it's going to be a great experience. That's what you will be offering to your patients when you own the area of logistics. I can't tell you many offices out there have let logistics take a back seat for far too long. They don't have a good handle on their procedures, inventory, and systems. This holds them back more than they could imagine. Patients can see and sense that there is a problem. They may realize that your office doesn't have their act completely together, or they may find your office so disorganized that they no longer have the level of trust that they should.

Owning it when it comes to logistics means you are going to put the focus on getting your procedures and protocol right. When you do that, you will see the benefits that come in terms of efficiency and productivity, as well as in the attitude of your team and patients. Everyone loves a well-organized office that is prepared, knows what to do, when to do it, and how to do it. That's putting the patient first and letting them know you have covered all the bases and are ready to provide them with the best care and convenience in your town.

"No business can succeed in any great degree without being properly organized."
- James Cash Penney

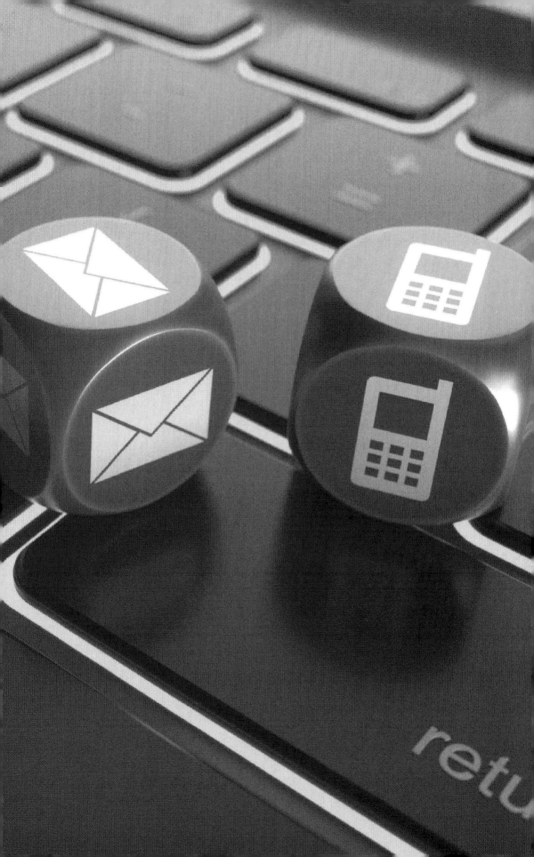

CHAPTER FOUR
COMMUNICATION

"You can have brilliant ideas, but if you can't get them across, your ideas won't get you anywhere." — Lee Iacocca

It doesn't matter how great a doctor you are if you don't have the means to communicate that to people. *Communication is the basis of what's going on in your practice.* It's the glue that will keep all of the pieces of the puzzle together. It's also the third of the 15 core areas that you can choose to own.

Owning communications is a great way to ensure that your practice has effective relationships with everyone it comes into contact with. From vendors and patients to your employees and referring dentists, there are no stones left unturned in the quest to provide effective communication.

Communication affects your practice in many more ways than you may even realize. It's much more than just making sure your receptionist offers a warm welcome to everyone who walks in the door. You want to do that, but beyond that there are ways you are handling, or not handling, communication in your office that can have a major impact on its overall well being.

The Many Impacts

How are you and your staff at talking with insurance companies? Believe it or not, this is a major area of communication that many orthodontic practices utterly fail. Whoever it is that is on the phone with them usually doesn't know what to say, what they need, and how to effectively ask for it. This is a problem, because you need to have a great line of communication with the insurance companies you deal with.

When we realized that there were communication problems with this area of our practice, we took measures to address it. As a result, we saw collections go through the roof. You can't possibly get the collections you need if the communication with those paying isn't what it should be. You can't wait around for the insurance companies to sort things out and improve communications on your behalf. Let's face it, it's probably not in their best interest. They make the payments, and the longer they can keep the money, the better it is for them and the worse it is for you. Effective communication can help close that gap like nothing else will.

How do you talk with referring doctors and how often do you communicate with them? What are your privacy practices like? I can tell you that after going through it painfully, those who are part of my private client group get everything handed to them on a silver platter, which includes my new HIPAA privacy training program for my employees. Here's a little secret for you – if you are not actually training your employees every six months with a documented privacy practices training program that's been certified, and you are not actually getting signatures and testing them and getting answers to the test every six months for every employee, then you are in violation of HIPAA privacy practices. Many people are not aware of this, but I know, because I've been through this and survived it all.

What we have used in the past for HIPAA and what we have in place now couldn't be further apart. They are like different planets and it's unbelievable. Maybe this is an area that you know you need to focus on. Or maybe it's your human resource practices that get you excited. Perhaps your spouse used to work in human resources and that got you interested and excited about that area. It doesn't matter which area it is, it just matters that you pick one and you own it.

Automation Perks

The good thing about owning the area of communication is that once you make the decision to own it and start covering all of your areas within it, you can actually automate a lot of it. In our office, for example, we automate all of the things that happen once a patient starts treatment. We do this so that we don't have to worry about things like insurance going missing, wondering who filed it, and trying to find the paper trail. Everything is automated. If you are

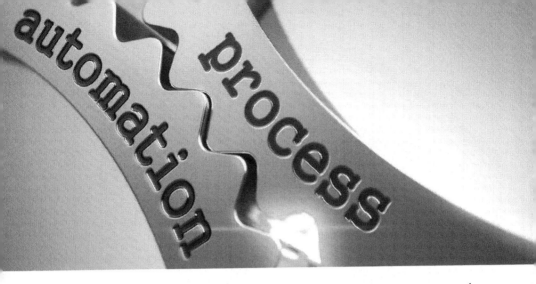

a client of ours and we recommend OrthoFi, and you are going to use it, they do it all for you, right? It's the same type of idea here. Who in your practice has the eye for owning communications?

Often times, practices don't realize how important owning their communication is until something happens. When something comes up missing, misunderstood, or people are left not knowing what procedure to follow, then they realize there is a gap in the communication that needs to be fixed. Those who own the area of communication look ahead to plan wisely so that all of the bases are accounted for and covered.

It may surprise you to learn that from our secret shopper data we found what I consider a scary little statistic. That is, many patients show up at your practice without their health history forms or without accurate data in the system. That's a communication problem that is downright embarrassing. It's horrible and it's something that should never happen. Owning the area of communication ensures that it won't. Communication is an area that may just get you excited.

Why Communication

If you are wondering why you should consider owning the area of communication, turn it around ask why you shouldn't. Every practice in the country is run with communications. We can't get much of anything done if we don't communicate effectively with our staff, patients, referring doctors, or anyone else we may come into contact with. Effective communication is essential for having a successful practice. With it, your office will run smoothly and there will be no guessing, chasing, and pointing of fingers. With it, everyone knows what the procedures are, and how everything works to take care of every patient who walks through the door.

It's not just communication that you are after when you decide to own this area. It's effective communication. There's a big difference in having communications that are effective and ones that are not. Without a doubt you have dealt with your fair share of poor communications over the years. Have you ever read some instructions on how to put something together, only to have no understanding of the process once you are done? That's because while there was communication, it wasn't at all effective. When communication is effective, there will be no questions or very few, because the information has been well thought out, planned, and shared.

There are many benefits to owning effective communication in your practice, and once you take this area on you will see a major difference. Having outstanding effective communication helps to create and maintain relationships with everyone. You will use your communication skills to help form and strengthen relationships with your patients, referring doctors, and your team members. Using effective communication practices with everyone you come into contact with at your office helps ensure that all needs are met and the people walk away with a good opinion of you and your practice. Even when you are not the one doing the communicating, owning this area will ensure that all of the communication coming out of your practice is effective, clear, and conducive to the goals and mission of your office.

Communication can also help lead to new ideas. When you give the people around you the ability to communicate their ideas with you, the sky is the limit on where your office can go. Without a doubt, some of them have some amazing ideas that are hidden away in their minds, just waiting for the right time to bring them out. When working on communication for your practice, you will find that there are new ideas that bubble up to the surface.

Owning communication is also great for your internal processes, as it will help your team to become more effective. When they can all communicate with one another, have written procedures to follow, and know exactly what is going to be done, by whom, and when, there will be a better synergy among your team. A team that doesn't talk to one another, or that doesn't get along isn't a team at all. And make no mistake, you want a team in your office. A team will work together, communicating and respecting one another, in order to help the overall mission of the practice. A team that communicates well together and with everyone they come into contact with will fare way better than those who don't.

A lack of communication leads to confusion, questions, disengagement, and a team that is unhappy. When you have an unhappy team, you will have an office that is not all it can and should be. Your practice can never reach the level of success that you would like to have without having a team that focuses on effective communication. It's an essential ingredient in every practice and one that is far too often overlooked. When your office owns the area of communications, you will remove the stress that comes from not being effective in this area. The questions dissolve, and take with them the stress and negative energy that usually accompany not having good communication around you.

Another reason to consider owning communication is that it helps to build trust and respect. This goes for those who work in your office, as well as for your patients, referral sources, vendors, and anyone else you may have dealings with. When you communicate well with each of these people, they will come to have more respect and trust for you and your office. That's always a good thing, because it's going to get you more dedicated employees, patients who love and rave about you, and doctors who want to refer more patients your way. Trust is the cornerstone of what we do, as every person we treat has to have a certain level of trust for us and the process. When you increase trust, you help to further build your practice. You may want to think of communication as the glue that holds your office together. It's an important and effective link between you, your employees, your patients, and your referring doctors. Pay no attention to that glue and it will deteriorate over time. But if you own it and give it attention, you will find that the bond is strengthened and does more to help provide a cohesiveness that you can't get elsewhere.

Body Language, Too

When discussing the importance of communication in your practice, we can't forget to look at the area of body language. The reason that this is important is because of the many secret shopper videos that I've watched. When you watch as many hours of these undercover videos as I have, you begin to see the things that need to be addressed that are often overlooked. But they can make a huge difference in the eyes of your patients, which makes it well worth exploring and addressing.

Imagine walking into a doctor's office where none of the employees even look up from their desk. You walk up to the reception window to check in and you are asked to sign in and take a seat, without the receptionist ever looking up at you. Instead, she is filing her nails, looking at a magazine, or is deep in conversation with another co-worker about a movie she watched the night before. If you are that patient, how welcome do you feel about an experience like that? Chances are, you don't feel like they appreciate the fact that you are there and you may even wonder if you are interfering with their conversation. It's not a good experience for the patient and it helps to create an image for your office that isn't one you likely want to send. But this happens more often than you can imagine, because there is no importance placed on communication.

Body language is all around us. It's something that we can't get away from if we are to see people in person. Believe me, it matters what your employees are doing when patients walk in the door. It matters if they are snapping gum and drinking a Big Gulp, or they are being attentive to every patient's needs. Body language counts in a big way and more so than most of us realize or may even want to care to believe. A drop in the shoulders, a roll of the eyes, or a tilt of the head, are all subtle signals that are sent that mean something to the person reading them. If you are going to own communication in your office, then you need to consider the area of body language, too.

While you don't want to make body language your focus, you do want to keep it in mind and if you see things going on in your office that need to be addressed then do so. Many times, people are not aware that their body language is sending the wrong kind of message until it is brought to their attention.

What it Includes
When you decide that the area of communication is the one that you will own, you will want to cover all your bases. Since this will be your area, you need to nail it like it's nobody's business. You will want to make sure that every area of

communication in your practice has been evaluated and addressed. You want to be the type of place that people say has the best service in town, so go the extra mile and stand out for how effectively you communicate in every area of your practice.

Some of areas you will want to ensure that you evaluate and plan for include your internal and external communications. This includes everything from employee newsletters and having an idea white board to finding ways to effectively communicate with those outside the office, too. Consider such communication tools as helpful articles that have been written by you that can be given to patients. These can offer everything from how braces can help beat bullying to the best snacks for those with braces. This communication with them will be helpful and they will appreciate it even if you never directly hear the feedback.

Good communication means you have procedures in place, so that everyone knows what to do in a variety of situations. It takes the guesswork out of the process, so people are not wondering who does what and how it's typically done. Your communications should include internal and external strategies. Don't forget to focus on public relations. Send out periodic press releases about what new services you offer, how you support your community and inform the media about local events you plan to attend.

Effective communication from your office can go a long way toward helping to position yourself as an expert in your community. You can do this by writing articles that you submit to local newspapers and magazines for publishing, as well as writing press releases that put ideas in front of reporters, so they will interview you for the stories they put together. Sending out a list of braces approved Halloween candy every October, for example, is communication that will get you some media attention and help identify you in the community as an expert.

Another important area that falls under owning communication for your practice is your social media efforts and online presence. Even if you are not someone who likes to use social media or goes online much, you better believe most of the families of your patients do. Many begin their search online for doctors, read reviews, and look for local information. You need to be there, effectively communicating with them at every turn. Owning this area of communication for your practice means that you will be using social media tools in a professional manner that offers helpful information, you respond to messages you receive in a timely manner, you address negative reviews or complaints that may be posted online, and that you keep your website fully updated.

In this day and age, you can't even think about not having a website for your practice. In fact, you need to have one that is not just there, but is great. It needs to offer all of the information potential and current patients may be in need of, and it needs to be easy to navigate. The last thing you want is people becoming frustrated by trying to visit your site that is down, difficult to load, or that doesn't offer them the information they are looking for. Owning communication in this area also means having your site developed with search engine optimization in mind, so that people will find it when doing searches for braces or Invisalign in your geographic area.

On our website, we try to offer effective communication and take it seriously. We have a resource section, where we have new patient forms, a variety of articles and videos that offer helpful information and address frequently asked questions, and we have a news section, so we can offer links to where we have been interviewed in the news, as well as books that we have published that are of interest to patients and their families.

Getting it Done

If you decide that communication it the area you want to own, great, you will never regret it. I also know that many people who consider this area are often overwhelmed. They see the many areas that need to be addressed with effective communication and, well, it kind of makes them want to run in the other direction. That's understandable if you feel that you alone have to take on the massive amount of work that is required to own this area, but it doesn't need to be that way.

There is a good chance that you have an employee who is great at communication and who would love to make this a part of their job. While you want to offer articles and have a great website, for example, you don't need to feel like you have to take on writing and learning how to do HTML so you can write code for your website. You just need to know how to go about hiring the people who can make each of those things happen for you. Being an amazing leader means that you know your limits and are willing to delegate, trusting people to take on and excel in various areas where their strengths lie. It's all about seeing what needs to be addressed and putting the right people in place to make it happen. Many of these things, as mentioned earlier, can be automated so that once it's in place you just keep it going. This works especially well with something like sending out new patient welcome packets. You have all of the communication materials in place, and then it becomes automated for our employees to get it sent out every time, on the dime, no excuses.

You also want to focus on keeping things simple. You don't need to overdo it or become too elaborate. Those you deal with appreciate simple communication that gets to the point and gives them the information they need. Find the places where you can address a situation, keep the solution simple, and automate it. Always remember your audience, so that the message is tailored to them and their needs, and have a plan so that you keep going with it.

Being a great communicator isn't all about what you say and the information you provide to others. It also means that you are a good listener, so you want you and your team to also focus on improving their listening skills. Patients will often tell you what they want or need, but we are not always listening.

Owning the area of communication means that as a leader in your practice, you realize how important it is that information be shared in an effective manner. You will be taking on the responsibility and setting the bar for how people in your practice should communicate with one another, with your patients, referral sources, internally, and externally. It's an important area of any business that can make a huge difference in how you are received. Owning it is deciding that communication is no longer going to take a back seat in your office.

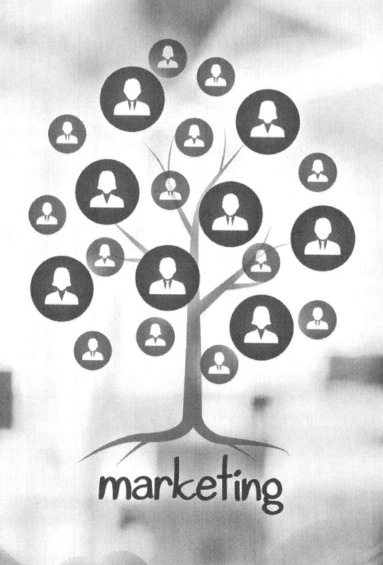

CHAPTER FIVE
MARKETING

"Marketing is a contest for people's attention." — Seth Godin

Marketing is something that is extremely important to every business on the planet, including every orthodontic practice. Yet many orthodontists haven't realized this or don't have a grasp of the vast importance that it makes in their practice. I've seen it all too often, where doctors don't have a clue as to how to go about effectively marketing their products and services. When this happens, you can't possibly reach the level of success that you'd like to reach.

When it comes down to it, it doesn't matter how great a doctor you are if you don't know how to tell people what you have to offer. It also doesn't matter how innovative and helpful the products and services you offer can be if you don't know how or take the time to let people know about them. You could have the best possible system for straightening teeth that there is, but if it remains hidden in a back office closet and nobody talks about it, you fail the patient, your team and yourself.

Marketing Counts

Marketing is an area that has brought us a lot of attention. We take it seriously and share our results with orthodontists all over the planet. There are some important questions to consider when it comes to your office's marketing efforts. For starters, how do you attract new patients and new referring doctors? How do you encourage referrals? What's your internal marketing system look like?

Maybe the idea of marketing, or even one particular area of marketing such as internal marketing, is something that gets you really excited. It doesn't matter if marketing is the one area that gets you excited or one particular area of it, you can choose to own the area of marketing. Do it better than anyone else in your market. Commit to doing it better than it's ever been done before. Become so efficient at marketing that it will make your competitors' heads spin. You want to be that great at marketing. You want to stand out as the practice that has nailed marketing, excels at it and leaves all others in the dust.

We do a ton of internal marketing, making up around 80% of our total marketing investment each month. This is probably a serious shocker to those on the outside who see all of the external marketing that we do, but in reality what they are seeing is a small portion of our overall effort. I'm known in my area for doing a lot of external marketing, but what we have owned in this area is our internal marketing practices.

Perfecting and Automating

What happens systematically when a patient says yes to treatment? This is an incredibly important area that you need to make a plan for so that you can maximize your efforts. Once someone agrees to treatment, there should be an experience that they then make their way through. It's important to play prospect, just like so many good companies do, such as Disney, Ritz-Carlton, Ferragamo, Audi, BMW, and Porsche. If you don't play prospect, see what shows up in the mail, see what shows up in your email, and see what shows up online following you around.

Through automation, the experience for each patient in our practice is consistent. This allows us to maximize the return on our marketing investment. We have also created the experience with our mission in mind, so that we take the time to market the right products and services to each and every patient. These unique offers are presented to the right patient at the right time, consistently. Years ago, our system was nearly impossible to manage and scale. Today, it has become second nature to everyone in the office, making it easier for our team to work together to help the patient navigate the perfect treatment experience. This creates a happier patient and a happier team because we've eliminated the guesswork and set clear expectations throughout the entire patient lifecycle.

At our practice, we know there is a right way and a wrong way for everything to happen. Disney calls this "Good show, bad show" and spends countless hours

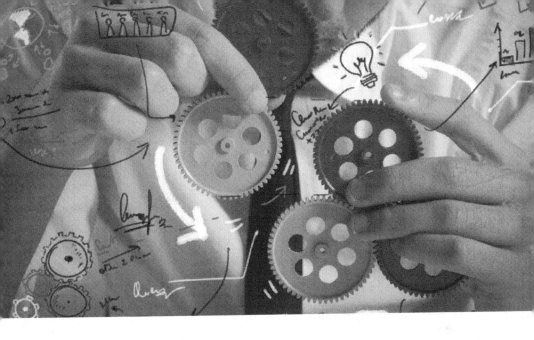

training their cast members the difference between doing it the wrong way and doing it the Disney way. This doesn't happen by accident. Remember, I've watched thousands of hours of secret shopper video, where we have observed what didn't happen, and realized what should have happened, with each patient. We have also studied extensively with the Disney Institute and Ritz Carlton Leadership to determine the best course of action in our practices. By owning it, our internal marketing has virtually been unstoppable. We have nailed it, but it's because we said we wanted to and then we put forth the effort and commitment to achieve our goals.

After you have covered all your bases, take the time to automate each area in your practice. When you automate, that's when the fun really happens. Everything gets done that needs to be done, your team will go through their day with less stress, and your practice will continue to grow with less effort and frustration. Leave no stone unturned in your quest to own the area of marketing. For example, we know that when patients were surprised with a caramel apple after getting their braces off, we saw referrals go up. We saw social media posts go up. We saw parents gushing about it in our office and online. We knew right there and then that we wanted that to happen every time someone got their braces off, so we automated the process and this happens every time now.

Taking the time to automate something as simple as making sure patients can have a caramel apple after their braces are off is beyond easy. Plus, the return on investment is incredible. Being able to surprise them with something like that puts a huge smile on their face, their parents' faces, and they can't wait to take a picture and post about it. Every time they do, it's someone else giving us a mention, rather than us giving ourselves one.

If you need help automating your marketing, call our friends at Ortho Marketing Done for You at 888-330-2566 or look them up on the web at OrthoMarketingDFY.com They are assisting our clients all over the world who want to take Burleson-Style marketing and automate it with powerful CRM software like InfusionSoft.

Targeting Your Audience

When it comes to marketing your practice, there are two main routes you can take. Those routes are external marketing and internal marketing. Both involve different angles and activities, but in the end they are both going to share information about your practice and help get more people to begin treatment. It is important to target your market, so that you always keep in mind who your campaign is for, whether it is something you are working on that will be seen externally or something that will be more internal.

As mentioned earlier, the majority of our marketing effort is placed on internal marketing. Once you watch as many secret shopper videos as we have, you see how important it is that you place an emphasis on internal marketing, but that doesn't mean you should ignore external marketing efforts. By owning marketing, you can certainly have a balance of the two that will give you the leverage you need to get more referrals through the door.

Targeting your marketing message, you may have efforts that are focused on reaching current and past patients, future patients, referring dentists, and even school nurses. One of the beautiful things about owning marketing is that there are many options and directions you can take with it. Whether you want to focus on owning one or two areas of marketing, or as many areas as you can organize and execute, there is a lot of variety. In the marketing world, it is important to always target your market so that your message is more effective and you have a higher return on investment.

External Marketing

The area of external marketing is one that you are likely going to be more familiar with. Most orthodontists are familiar with this type of marketing, which focuses on getting your practice name and brand image out to the public. There are numerous ways that it can be done today, giving you plenty of options to consider when putting together your plan of action.

Some of the areas of external marketing you will want to consider include:

 Social media. While this also falls under the area of communications, it is also an important tool in the area of marketing. Most adults use some form of social media, with Facebook being the most popular for adults in U.S. at the time of this writing. Your social media marketing efforts will include those caramel apple shots, as well as offering helpful tips, content, and even throwing in some contests here and there. Your online marketing efforts need to go beyond just using social media, however. You also need to include such areas as online advertising and using search engine optimization on your website, so that it helps it to show up when people do searches for braces information in your area. You may even use social media for helping to have referral contests. The options are endless.

 Advertising. This is the one area that you are likely familiar with. Most orthodontists have taken the time to do some advertising by placing ad in a magazine or other such publication. What most of them have missed the mark on, though, is making sure that their advertising efforts are effective. To improve your return on investment and just make sure you are not throwing money down the drain, it is imperative that you track your advertising dollars and determine how many leads they bring in. Adjust it where necessary, so that your dollars are not wasted. Your goal here is to get the most bang for your buck, but you will only know if you accurately track the source of each new patient.

 Content. One of the most effective ways you can market your practice is through helpful content. Your mission here is to become an effective content king. The kind of content I'm referring to here are the things we have focused on in our practice. This includes helpful articles, books, and papers that readers will want and will gain insight from. The key here is that it has to be interesting and helpful to them. A big mistake that people make is to turn their content efforts into something that is overly technical or to make it all about marketing themselves. That's a route that will get your content quickly ignored. Make it something a parent will want to read and keep the marketing to a byline at the end of the piece or something subtle. For example, articles on the best snacks for kids with braces, or foods to avoid, or when kids should first see a dentist, are all helpful topics that are evergreen. They are always of interest to readers and never go out of style. Your external marketing will also focus on where to place your content for maximum exposure.

Mailings. There are marketing materials that should be sent out to people, such as a new welcome packet for new patients, birthday cards for your patients, and other notes here and there. Maybe it's a one-year anniversary of someone being a patient, or perhaps you heard they just earned the Little League MVP award, or maybe it's sending out handwritten thank you notes every time someone refers someone to your office. There are many opportunities for sending out a mailing. Plus, they can all be automated.

Testimonials. Your marketing efforts should include gathering some testimonials from your happy patients. This can be done in the form of written testimonials, pictures and one quote, or they can be videos. You can even try a few different ways so that you have a variety. People enjoy hearing what others in the community have to say about their experience with their treatment. Post them on social media channels, your website and other appropriate places. Manage your online reviews. Whether on your Facebook page or on other review sites, stay on top of reviews and address any that may be less than great.

Image. Make no mistake – your brand image is part of your marketing efforts. If you have already taken a look at your logo and image, great, but if it's something you have been ignoring then it's time to take a serious look at it. You must have an image that represents your company well and it must be used effectively in your marketing efforts.

Internal Marketing

This is the area, as mentioned, that most orthodontists seem to fall short on. They usually overlook how important it is to growth and referrals. Internal marketing is what you are doing on the inside of your practice, so it's the efforts that are made within the walls of your business. It can mean the efforts that you make to sell additional services and products to those patients who come in through your doors, and there should absolutely be a process in place for this. But there's something even more important that internal marketing means, and that's the area that I want to focus on here.

Internal marketing can give you an infinite amount of referrals. It's directly correlated to the overall culture of your practice and what you share with your employees. Do you share your vision with them and ensure they know how you want every patient treated? If not, then your internal marketing will fall short and it's going to cost you. A lot.

Secret shopper videos show that when practices fall short in the area of internal marketing they have a team that isn't cohesive. They have a culture in the office that is not conducive to referrals and giving people a reason to say great things when they leave your office. Most orthodontists provide adequate customer service. The experience is fine but not great. Most offices really don't give the patient a reason to talk about them.

We have all heard stories about exceptional customer service at Disney. These stories are intentionally shared from cast member to cast member and from guest to guest. This isn't by mistake. Disney makes it a point to share stories worth sharing. Crawling through broken glass for your customers when something goes wrong, remembering their name, treating them to unexpected surprises and small gifts. How are you encouraging your team and your patients to share the stories worth sharing?

Your mission when it comes to internal marketing is to share your vision with your team and get them on board with it. Once you do that, you will multiply your energy working toward that goal, because each of them will be an ambassador for your brand. Get your team on board with what you want your patient experience to be like and they will help convert people to starting treatment, as well as get you more referrals. When people love their experience at your office, they are going to tell other people about it. Word of mouth marketing like this is worth its weight in gold.

Some of the ways you will want to focus on internal marketing include, but are not limited to:

- Ensure that the person answering your phones has the right training and personality for providing great patient service. This means helping to get questions answered and diligently finding appointment times that meet the patient's needs. Remember, this is the voice of your practice, so it is important that this person is on board with your mission and knows how to go about providing excellent patient care.

- Set the tone in your office starting with the moment a patient walks in the door. They should be warmly greeted and the office should look great and be comfortable. This area was already discussed more in length, but it is also part of internal marketing.

- Train your team to check on patients to ensure they are kept comfortable throughout their entire appointment. Every patient needs to feel that your office cares about them and sees them as more than just another person getting treatment in the books.

- Let employees know how they should interact with patients. While this may seem like something that is so basic that they should already know it, I can assure you from the videos we have seen that there are plenty of people who do not.

- Create a patient experience at each stage, including when they begin treatment, during treatment, and when they have completed treatment. The new patient experience is crucial to every practice so that people start off on the right foot from the start. The patient experience is something everyone needs to be aware of so that it is automated and there is consistency.

There must be an emphasis placed on building relationships. People refer other people when they trust the work that your office provides. Trust is built on relationships, and your employees need to be aware of this and on board with it completely. When you focus on owning your internal marketing, you will be encouraging better performance among your team, you will improve engagement, and everyone will become more committed to growth.

Owning It

From the new patient experience to ensuring your team is a cohesive one that is on board with what it means to provide excellent patient care, internal marketing works. It means spending more time looking inward, to make improvements in the office and employees, so that the overall experience for the patient is smoother, more enjoyable, and something they will want to recommend to others.

When you choose to own it, marketing will become second nature to you even though at this point it may seem like there is a lot to focus on. When you own a particular area, however, you will become an expert in it and do it better than any other practice in your area. Owning it means you will become known for your external and internal advertising. While many people will see your efforts on the outside, as they do ours, those who step into your office will know and feel the internal marketing even more.

Marketing is all about taking what you do and making sure that people know about it, especially those who would be candidates for treatment or know someone who is. It's finding clever ways to consistently put your information and name out there to shape how people see your office. This is done from the inside looking out, and from the outside looking in, and both areas should get some attention, even if you choose to own only one area more than the other, as we do.

Just as Lee Iacocca said, you may have the best ideas in the area of orthodontics, but if you don't put forth the effort to let people know and experience it, then it will essentially mean nothing. Owning the area of internal marketing ensures those ideas are effectively disseminated.

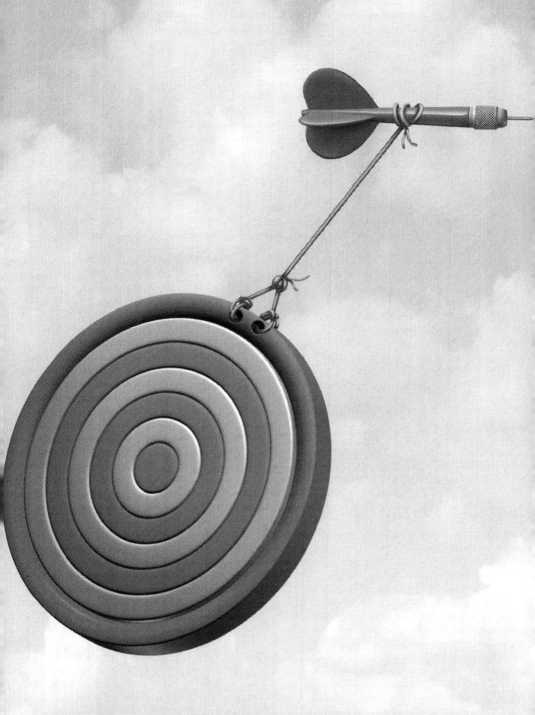

CHAPTER SIX
SALES

"A goal is a dream with a deadline." – Napoleon Hill

When many people hear the word "sales," they tend to become anxious. That's because the word has often become synonymous with high-pressure tactics that tend to turn people off. We often think of the used car salesman, the solicitor who rings our doorbell during dinner, or the person who talks you into something you soon realize you never needed in the first place. While all of these people do exist and I'll be the first to agree that they can tax the nerves, it's not what I'm referring to when I want you to focus on owning sales.

We live in a world that is driven by sales, so even the person who thinks they are not selling something is doing exactly that at the end of the day. Every business on the planet is selling something. Every employee is selling something as well – their human capital. *We all have something to sell, but we don't all have good sales skills.* The good news is that this is something you can change. In fact, selling is an area that you can own and excel in if you decide you want to.

Sales Matter
In the field of orthodontics, many people don't like to think of what they are doing as sales. Yet that's exactly what you are doing. Let me explain why before you start squirming around at the thought of being a salesperson. Sales, simply put, are the revenue that is earned from your services and products. Every time someone begins treatment you have gotten a sale. We may not go around calling it that, but that's what it is, and it's not a bad thing. In fact, sales are critical to our practice's success.

Sales give you the means to pay your employees' salaries, pay your overhead, and take home a salary of your own. Sales are what helps you reach your company goals and become more successful. *Sales will make or break your practice and it's just that simple.* With a steady stream of sales, your practice will be successful, but without them you can't exist. Now that we have gotten that out of the way and you feel comfortable thinking about the fact that you are selling something, we can delve into this topic even more.

As you read through the ideas that you can own in this book, you may shy away from some, thinking you can't possibly imagine your practice owning that particular area. That's OK. As I have mentioned, you don't need to own all of these areas, but you do need to pick one of them to own and own it like no others in your area. You have to become known for it, excel at it, and make it look easy. You have to find that one area that you really love and make it yours. You need to take it, own it, and go light the world on fire with it.

Sales is a great area to own, because it's directly tied to your company's success and is what you strive for every year. Maybe you will want to own focusing on new patient conversion, like a client who recently sent me a very nice testimonial letter. What would a conversion rate of 85-90% look like for your practice? Maybe you are the best at getting referrals and maybe you are really good at just talking with patients and saying "Hey, we love people like you. What friends can you send to us? Who do you know that would love to improve their smile and be a great fit for our office?"

It's not just about saying that to people and it's not for everyone. But there are people who are comfortable saying something like that, because they have owned this area. When you choose to own the area of sales, you have to be comfortable saying things like that and in looking for ways to bring in more referrals and increase your conversion rates. Not only do you have to be looking for and willing to introduce ways to do that, but you have to be committed to doing this on an ongoing basis.

Some of the things you will want to consider when you own the area of sales are how you go about adding new services, whether or not adding in pediatric dentistry would be a good move, and could you be really, really good at

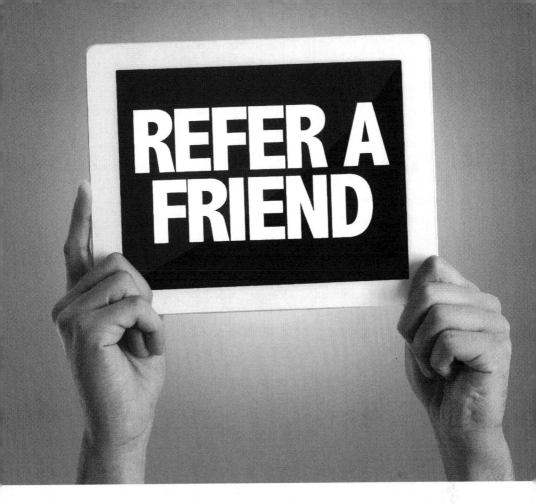

ensuring that when a patient gets their braces off that the next kid in treatment is started very quickly? What would excelling in these areas look like for your practice? I can tell you what it would look like, because these are things that we do already, and they have given us incredible leverage in our market.

The Focus

When it comes to owning sales, the two most important things you want to focus on are referrals and conversion rates. The more referrals you get, the more people who are going to walk through your doors. Every person is an opportunity to sell your services, which is where conversion comes in. When you focus on these two areas: setting goals and tracking to see if you are hitting the mark, you will do wonders for your practice. Referrals and conversion rates are so important that they could be stand-alone books all on their own.

Referrals are the backbone of your practice and you need a lot of them, a steady flow of them, in order to keep growing your practice. They can come from word-of-mouth sources, area dentists and hygienists, and they can come from others in the community. Referrals can come from numerous places and it's important for you to track the ones that you get. The best possible way to know what is working and what's not is to track every referral. Far too often, orthodontists don't track their referrals, so they have no idea which of their efforts are working or who their top referrers are in order to tap them for more and reward them.

If you don't already have a great referral system in place, you will absolutely need to have one if you decide to own the area of sales. The right referral system will keep a continuous flow of new patients coming in through your door, giving you plenty of people to focus on converting to treatment. While many people get a little anxiety over the thought of putting a referral system into place, it's not rocket science, and it is something you can do. The great thing about it, too, is that once it is in place it is automated for the most part. It will continue to chug along, doing what it does to bring people in, and most of it will be so automated that you will no longer feel like the system is much work at all.

Your referral system is going to target several areas, including word-of-mouth referrals, dentists and hygienists in your area and others in the community who may be able to send people your way, such as school nurses and pediatricians. There are plenty of things you can do to automate the act of reaching out to each of these sectors in order to keep the door to referrals open. Let's look at some of the main areas that you will want to focus on when creating your referral system.

Word of Mouth

It's hard to get better than someone else referring people to your office. While it is one thing for you to advertise and tell people why they should choose your office, it will never be the same or quite as convincing as someone else they trust telling them that. *When someone they trust, a friend or acquaintance, tells them that they should give your office a call it's a powerful testimonial.* The person is essentially vouching for you and your office, and the other person is more likely to end up getting treatment with you, because they trust getting the referral from someone they know.

One of the most important keys to a great referral system is identifying your top referrers and then treating them like royalty. Find out who sends the most patients your way. Thank them for it and show your gratitude. Give them even more reasons to continue sending people to you. You can only achieve this type of relationship with your best referral sources if you track accurately. Teach your team to accurate track where every referral comes from. Create an automated system to thank them promptly. You want to reach out to every referral source and thank them every time you get a new referral. You can do this by sending a hand-written note, or you can surprise them with a gift card to their favorite restaurant. You should also plan to have some VIP referral parties throughout the year, where you shower them with gratitude and recognition.

In order for people to want to tell others about your office, you must provide an amazing experience. Do you think that so many people would talk to others about their Disney experience if it were just OK? Not a chance. Disney has made the experience so great that people can't wait to tell others about it. They post pictures, write up online reviews, and go home telling everyone about it. What happens next is that some of those they tell begin wanting to plan their trip to Disney. The same thing happens with the new Apple iPhone. When the iPhone gets a new model not everyone is in need of a new phone, but once they hear others talking about it they just have to have it, and off they go to get it.

There is one major rule when it comes to getting word-of-mouth referrals. You cannot be boring. Nobody talks about or refers people to boring. People refer their friends and family to those who are anything but boring. They refer them to those who go above and beyond, to those who surprise them and those who excite them. This means that you have to have a great patient experience. If you do, people will talk about it, and you will get referrals from it. If you don't, then there won't be much talk. Start by making a list of everything that irritates people when they visit a doctor's office. One by one, find a way to eliminate every single item on your list. This is why our offices are open late. This is why we are obsessed with running on time and why we got rid of our front desk. It's why we finance the way we do, market the way we do and interact with our patients the way we do. We made a list years ago of everything that pisses patients off and we set out to systematically destroy every item on the list. We led an insurgency against the status quo and our patients have been rewarding us ever since.

Dental Referrals

At this point, you should already have a good idea of who your top referring dentists are. If you don't, that is something that has to change immediately. You should know where every dentist is who has referred people to you. Make a point to build a relationship with them and their office, so they will continue to send referrals your way. Get to know them, stop in once in a while to say hello, send them a thank you note, order a pizza party to be delivered on a Friday afternoon for lunch, do things throughout the year that will keep you on their mind and in their good graces.

While you want to build a relationship with the dentists at each of these places, it's not only the dentist you want to focus on. Be sure to let your personality shine to the entire office, including to the hygienists, as they also speak with people who may ask them for an orthodontist they would refer in the area. This may happen both inside the office and while they are at a party on a Friday night. Since people know they are in the dental field, they will feel comfortable asking them for who they would turn to in the field. They trust their opinion and you want to be a part of the advice that they offer to the person.

In strengthening the dental office referral rate, you will also want to keep them stocked with the referral materials they need. Often, people want to refer someone to your office, but they may not know the best way go about doing it. Owning this area means you will help make that easier for them. You can do this by providing them with some good content they can keep on hand that they can give out to their patients who they may want to refer to you. Write a book or a few articles that answer common questions you receive as a specialist from concerned parents. They trust their dentist, so getting the information and referral from them will help increase your conversion rate.

Other Referrals

Word of mouth referrals and those coming from local dentists' offices are not the only source of referrals there are, although they will likely make up the bulk of them. There are some other areas that you can get referrals from that are usually untapped resources for orthodontists. *Those who have a great referral system in place will tap into these other areas and will get creative with the many ways they can find ways to get their foot in the referral door.*

Places to consider for other referral sources include pediatrician offices, school nurses, and parenting groups. Each of these entities offers a way for you to meet those who may need your services. Get to know these people who are in the positions and give them materials that make sense for their audience. For example, if you are going to focus on a local pediatrician's office and want to build that relationship, have an article made all about how to take care of a child's teeth, or what to do if you suspect your child may need braces. With your info on the article, having it placed in their office is going to help get you referrals from the parents who frequent their office.

The same goes with the school nurses. You can meet with them and supply them with some helpful tools to care for those kids who come to their office with some common minor braces issues. With the schools and parenting groups, you can inquire about becoming a community partner, where you may even get the chance to speak to the group, do demonstrations, and send home information. Keep in mind that every opportunity to send home information is a window of opportunity. Make it count by giving them helpful information that is targeted to that specific audience. You have a short time span to grab their attention and for it to be meaningful to them.

Relationship Building

When you think about owning sales, you most likely just picture all of the numbers. Yes, it's important to know the numbers, such as your referral rates, conversion rates, and how many people are getting treatment per year, among other things. But there is one huge thing you have to focus on that is even more important and will aid you in getting all the numbers that you want. It's relationship building, and in order to be good at sales you have to put an effort into building relationships.

The type of selling that we do is dependent upon great relationship building. People buy from those who they trust, and they refer people to those who they trust. Trust is the common theme and you can't have trust without a relationship. This means you need to focus on getting to know people. I mean the type of stuff that goes beyond just saying hello. It means getting to know their name and using it, it means knowing that they like the Baltimore Orioles, and that their son plays second base in the local little league.

When you get to know people, asking questions and sharing some things about yourself, you will be building a relationship. Those relationships are going to bring in a steady stream of referrals. It's all about being nice, being fun, being interesting, and being interested in others. It's easy to do and it's actually good for your health, so you get a bonus there. Plus, the relationship building is something that can be partially automated and it's something that others in your office can help do. It can be a team effort so that the office has a great relationship with a referring dental office, as well as providing an excellent patient experience so that every patient walks out wanting to tell others how great your office is.

Pediatric Dentistry

One effective way to get a lot of referrals is to consider adding pediatric dentistry to your practice, as we did. This is a great way to help focus on sales, because you already have the patients coming to your office. Those who are candidates for treatment will already be comfortable getting treatment right there with you and your staff. You will need to determine if the cost is worth the return on investment, but it's an excellent option to consider.

When you add pediatric dentistry to your orthodontic practice, you will be providing the public in your area with a family-centered office that offers a comprehensive approach to dental care. From the youngest of patients to those who need braces, you can handle it all right at your office. It can be a great way to help improve access to such care in your community, and help to increase your overall revenue at the same time, creating a win-win situation.

Pediatric dentists have a specialty of their own. They have been trained to work with the group of patients who just so happen to be the ones who are your target market. It only makes good sense to get them comfortable with your office, so that if they are a candidate for orthodontic care you will take care of it. Even if they are not, you will still be helping to improve your revenue, provide the community with additional pediatric dental care, and will have that many more people who are familiar with your office who can be referral sources out on the streets.

Owning It

Everyone who has their own practice should be interested in the area of sales. Owning it is a solid way to help your business reach the level of success that you want. Owning it means that you become comfortable reaching out and tapping into all of the ways that you can help to increase your sales, including your referral rates and conversion rates.

If you choose to own the area of sales, you must focus on creating a great referral system. You must focus on the inside and how patients perceive your office. This is how you create an amazing patient experience that gets people talking. It means your entire staff must be on board with delivering the experience and being committed to your vision.

Henry Ford knew how to build a great product. He perfected his cars over time to create something that he knew could be useful to many. Had he shied away from the area of sales, we likely wouldn't know his name and he surely wouldn't have left the legacy that he did. As an orthodontist, you have a skill that people need and want. Selling yourself, your practice and those skills and abilities is a must. If you own it, you can define what you want to do, what your goals are and you can put the wheels in motion to make it happen.

Owning it when it comes to the area of sales means that you will stop at nothing to do what it takes to create the systems that are needed to grow your practice to where you want it to be. A goal may be a dream with a deadline, but when that deadline includes revenue goals it always helps to be an expert in the area of sales.

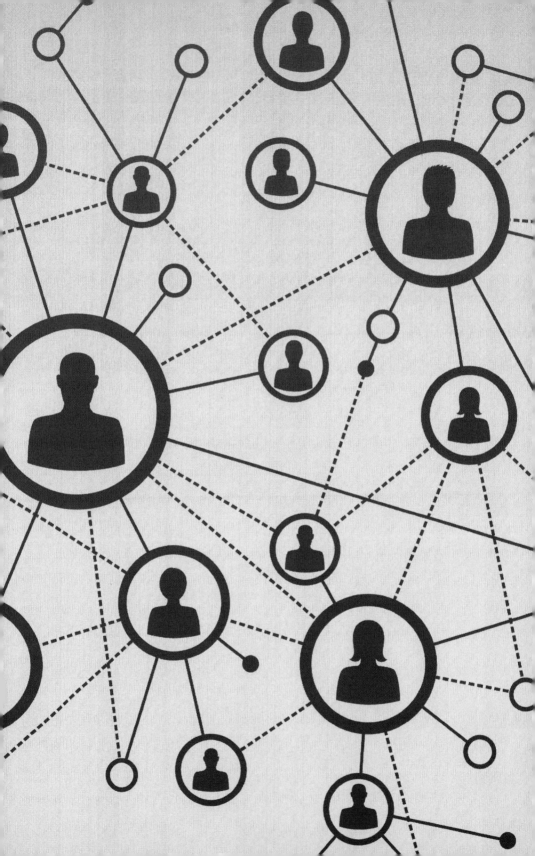

CHAPTER SEVEN
NETWORKING

"You can make more friends in two months by becoming interested in other people than you can in two years by trying to get other people interested in you." - Dale Carnegie

Networking is a term that is thrown around a lot in the business world, and for good reason. Most people who are successful in business or who are good leaders understand that there's something to networking that will help them get ahead. Not only can it help a business get ahead, but it can also open the door to many opportunities that may otherwise never come your way. Choosing to own the area of networking means that it's time to start mingling more than you have most likely been doing, and learning how to make the most of your efforts.

I've worked with many orthodontists around the world who fly to Kansas City for consulting services. While I share advice and strategies to help these doctors grow, I also learn a great deal from these consultations. I learn what they are doing. I see what's working and what's not, but more importantly I learn what they are ignoring entirely. Networking is one of those areas. It's largely ignored by most orthodontists and that presents a tremendous opportunity for those who take it seriously.

From what I have seen, we as orthodontists tend to do a lot of networking when we first open our practice. After that, once we start getting some patients come through the door, we tend to forget all about networking and the benefits that it can provide. I recall that when we first opened our doors, I was doing what I refer to as bootstrap marketing, which is literally pounding the pavement, knocking on doors, delivering cupcakes to local dentist offices, and shaking as many hands as possible. I had the time on my hands to be able to do that. After all, I didn't really have any patients at the time.

Back in 2006, we started with just one patient in our first month. That left me with a lot of time to engage in getting out and networking with local dentists and hygienists. Fast forward to today, and we have 11,000 active patients. There's a huge difference, and obviously I no longer have the time to personally pound the pavement to focus on networking. But that doesn't mean that we don't do it, because it's just the opposite. We actually do a lot of area networking. The key is putting someone in your practice into the position. Having a public relations coordinator is a huge asset, and one that will provide your office with a great return on investment if it's done correctly.

Do you have someone in your office who goes out and shakes hands, sits elbow-to-elbow, knee-to-knee, and talks to people? That's exactly what you need if you are going to own the area of networking. You need someone whose job it is to represent your practice, going out to talk with the dentists and hygienists, among others, who will be key players in being able to refer people to your office.

Networking Defined

Networking is more than just meeting people. It's actually a lot more than that. It's about the relationships you make with the people you meet. Anyone can meet people, shake hands, and exchange business cards. But that's not networking, and without doing things to cultivate that relationship it won't go much further than that. You are probably familiar with this scenario. You have made the introduction, the business card is promptly filed away, and then you don't do much else with the connection beyond that.

Owning the area of networking is going to drastically change all that. It's going to make those connections a major goal within your practice. There is a good chance that you don't have the time to go out and make all of the necessary connections that are needed to own networking and be great at it. You will need to have someone in your practice who will be great at carrying the mission out on your practice's behalf.

Networking is about building relationships. It goes beyond just simply making someone's acquaintance. It is the art of turning those acquaintances

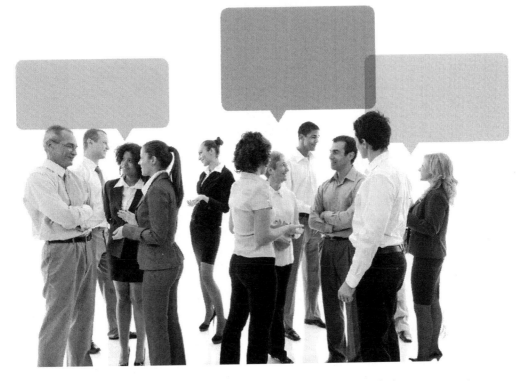

into relationships. These are people who may be able to help your practice by sending you lots of referrals over the year, so you have a vested interest in building good relationships with them.

Relationships are things that are built on a mutual trust and interest. When you take the time to get to know your point of contact, you will be cultivating a relationship. Maybe it starts with taking cupcakes to their office, but as it progresses you are mutually sharing information. You want to get to know the person beyond just whether or not they can send you some referrals. You want to know who their favorite hockey or baseball team is, what their favorite restaurant is, and that they still watch "Seinfeld" reruns every Saturday night. The more you know about this person and can connect them on a personal level, the stronger your relationship will become.

The people who you will be networking with should find the relationship to be mutually beneficial. The last thing you want is to be some sorry sap who just goes around contacting people to see what kind of referrals they can get that month. People see right through that, feel they are being used and will most likely not give the referrals you are seeking. On the other side, if you take the time to build strong and trusting relationships that are built on a mutual respect and interest, you will stand to gain many referrals and possibly some good friends and colleagues to boot.

By focusing on relationship building, you will also be surrounding your practice with positivity. Networking focuses on keeping the lines of communication open, and as Dale Carnegie points out, it shouldn't all just be about you and your practice. It's imperative that whoever is doing your public relations work gets to know the people by asking them questions and showing interest in them and their lives. That interest needs to be genuine, too, because people will see right through someone who is fake and trying to suck up just for the sake of getting referrals.

Keep relationship-building in mind and things should go well. Doing things to build and strengthen relationships is the name of the game when it comes to owning the area of networking.

The Many Benefits

There are many benefits that can come from networking that has been done right. The most important one for your practice is that you will most likely get referrals out of it. In order to grow your practice, maintain it, and reach the level of success you want, you will always need a steady supply of referrals coming your way. That can only be achieved with investing in relationships so that people will send others your way. Remember, people like to refer people to those they trust. If they have only met you and exchanged business cards, there is no trust there. The relationship hasn't been cultivated and they would probably have to be kind of desperate to want to start sending all of their referrals your way. Maybe they don't like the other orthodontist in the area at all and they have been waiting for someone else to walk through the door. Beyond that, you won't get much out of just that superficial meeting.

Take the time to grow a relationship, on the other hand, and you will end up getting many referrals. They will grow to know and trust you, and want to send their patients your way. They will feel good helping you out, as well as feel comforted knowing that their patients are in good hands. Their own reputation is on the line when it comes to making referrals. If they make poor ones and people are left unhappy, then it won't reflect well on them. Those they refer need to be happy with their treatment and service, and if they are then it will reflect well on the dentist who referred them to you.

The networking relationships you make can lead to more opportunities and additional connections. You never know what type of opportunities are going to emerge because of the relationships you cultivate with people. Perhaps you get invited to speak at a conference, be interviewed for a news story, or one dentist vouches for you to another, who begins sending referrals your way. The additional connections that the networking efforts lead to can always pay off, helping your office to become more visible and help you stand out in a crowded market.

Building reputable connections also helps to get your office more active in the community. As an orthodontist, you want to show people that you didn't open your doors to just take their money. You are someone who is part of the community. You care about the community and the connections you have within it. Being a part of the community, including reaching out to others in it to provide a mutually beneficial relationship, is going to help your practice to grow. That type of activity strengthens the position you have within the community. Trust me when I say that people are paying attention and they notice and appreciate those who have a tight-knit relationship with others in the community.

Another good opportunity that comes from owning the area of networking is that you can work on shared goals. That's where making the relationship mutually beneficial comes into play. Everyone has goals, whether it be business or personal, and when we can all share in helping each other to achieve them we will strengthen our own position as a result. In other words, when you help others in your area, it will come back to you in a variety of ways and bring good things that help you, too.

Networking with others can also help keep you up on the trends and provide you with new ideas. You may hear a lot of things, and most of them don't interest you in the slightest. But if you can get a couple of new and exciting ideas out of it then it is worth the effort, because new ideas can go a long way toward motivating, inspiring, and creating something great. Networking opens the door to a variety of people, each with their own experiences and ideas, which is going to be a positive thing.

Taking Charge

I get that you probably don't have the time to go rub elbows with all of the area dentists, hygienists and others who may be able to send you referrals. If you did, then you wouldn't have the time to take care of patients. While it's a great idea for you to work on cultivating the networking relationships you have the time for, you won't personally have the time that it takes to own this area doing it on your own. There's no reason you can't have someone in your office master this area on behalf of your practice.

The key in having someone else handle this is in making sure you pick the right person for the job. It's such an important position, especially if this is the area you choosing to own, that you can't put it in just anyone's hands. You have to be diligent in ensuring that the right person tackles this project on your behalf. So how do you know you have the right person? Well, you want to go for the person with the right personality. The person who is in charge of this should be someone who is energetic, happy, positive, and has an all-around outgoing and great personality. That's where these relationships start, after all, is with a great genuine personality.

The person in this position should be someone who is creative, a good speaker and communicator, has a business sense, and the ability to get along well with other people. Before filling this position with someone who has experience on paper, look more at personality. Many of the most successful companies out there, such as Google and Apple, hire for attitude and personality, rather than someone's experience. You can teach someone how to maintain a contact management database, but you can't teach someone to have a great attitude that people are automatically drawn to.

You may already have this person in your office and you just need to make some adjustments to have this become part of his or her job. If you don't have someone in the office that can take this on, then hire someone, even on a part time basis, so that their focus is on owning this area for your practice. If this is the area that you choose to own, the expenses involved in having this person, provided you have the right person in the position, will be worth the return on investment.

This person's job, whether it's their sole duty or it's a part of another job they do within the office, is to keep your office on the radar. Not only will they keep your office on the radar, but they will also do some serious relationship building, which will lead to a lot of referrals coming your way. Whether it's dropping off cupcakes, popping in to say hello, or sending a gift on the hygienist's birthday, all of this and more will be the job of the person you put in charge of this task.

Ways to Effectively Network

As mentioned, most people think of networking as simply shaking hands and exchanging business cards. Not much else happens beyond that. Well, that's not effective networking and there's very little if anything that will result from that type of connection. Although the connection has been made, there's no relationship that has been built, so there's no reason for it to go any further. Only when you go far beyond that will you reap the benefits of doing so, and if you are going to own it, then you have to commit to going far beyond that mediocre introduction. Your practice is counting on it.

Effective networking starts with an introduction, but there is an effort put in on a regular basis to turn that connection into something more than a business card tossed into a desk drawer. The last thing you want is for that card to be tossed into a drawer and for your office to be largely forgotten about. The dentists and hygienists in your area are referring people to someone, so if not you, then whom? You want to do what you can to make it your office they are referring people to, and that takes more than just a simple business card exchange.

For starters, you want to seek out those for whom it would make sense to put forth the extra networking effort. This is going to include the area dentists, hygienists, school nurses, pediatricians, and health reporters. You may also want to investigate to see if you have a popular mommy blogger in your area who has a great following of local moms. If so, add that person to your list to get to know, because chances are the parents following the blogger respect their opinion and will go to her for referral advice. You want to be on her mind when people come asking about local orthodontic offices.

All of these people represent areas where you will gain referrals if you are engaged in effective networking. Many people seek out only the local dentists, and don't get me wrong, they are absolutely important. However, they are not the only route to getting referrals and you don't want to overlook the others.

Consider how many children your local pediatrician sees each year. Many of them visit for annual and school physicals. Parents respect their doctor's opinion and may ask for advice about orthodontics, or the doctor may offer it if they can see there may be a problem that needs to be evaluated.

The school nurse also sees many children each year, as does the hygienist. Don't forget about the key people who are in the dentist's office who can become a referral source for your practice. If this is the area you will choose to own, you will want to get creative with it and go deep. Focusing only on the local dentists offices is just scratching the surface. There are a lot of other referral resources that are largely untapped that you can add to your area of focus. Tap them and you never know how far it will go and what it will bring your way.

It's important to note that this will not be a relationship where you are just expecting to get from each of these people. While you do want to get referrals from them, you can't just focus on that. The best relationships in the world are built on a mutual respect and give and take. If they feel that your interest only lies with what they can do for you and how they can help grow your business, then it likely won't be a long-lasting relationship. You need to find ways to do for them and help them, too. The effort needs to be mutual. Find ways that you can help their office or them personally, so that you are giving something back. Perhaps you can send some referrals their way, or you can provide continuing education experiences and other practice-building tools. Leave them feeling satisfied, rather than like they are being used only to get referrals.

The easiest way to begin building a relationship with others, whether it is with the pediatrician in the office across the street or it's with someone you want to become friends with, is to show interest in them. When you show interest in other people, you will engage them and begin to build the foundation of a relationship. Each time you meet or have contact it can't all be about you, your office, and what they can do for you.

Owning It

When you decide to own the area of networking, you also have to take full responsibility for all first impressions. They count more than most people realize. In fact, the Society for Personality and Social Psychology reports that even someone's appearance can override what someone has heard about a person. They also report that appearance overrides facts, and that good first impressions must be done in person, not virtually.

First impressions form opinions that stick with people, even when they have heard facts and information that differs from their impression. It gets ingrained in our brains and those first impressions are very difficult to overcome, even as time goes on and there are additional chances for communication. This makes it essential that whoever is put in charge of your networking knows the importance of first impressions and will strive to always make a great first impression. The person needs to be friendly, confident, prepared, be a good listener, and be dressed appropriately. As much as we'd like to think that we don't judge books by their cover, that's exactly what the research shows that we consistently do.

Owning networking will put you in a position to have your office build and maintain great relationships with those who can send you a steady stream of referrals. It can be a fun mission that gets your office noticed, respected, loved, and can help you become wildly successful if you own it in the right way.

"Networking is more about 'farming' than it is about 'hunting'. It's about cultivating relationships." - Dr. Ivan Misner

---

CHAPTER EIGHT
PSYCHOLOGY

"If there is any one secret of success, it lies in the ability to get the other person's point of view and see things from that person's angle as well as from your own." – Henry Ford

Henry Ford knew exactly how important it was to understand other people's points of view. Without this skill, he may have never achieved the amazing success that he did in his lifetime. He revolutionized how things are made, perfecting the assembly line, and he gave people the ability to own a vehicle. You could say that he had a good understanding of psychology and he used it to his advantage.

You don't have to be Sigmund Freud to use psychology to your advantage in the field of business. Every highly successful business out there has used it to some extent in order to tap into their customers' minds, sell them something, sell them more, and to make a connection with them. That's just good business. It's smart business. And it's something that every orthodontist can do.

Psychology Defined

The more you realize how you can use the idea of psychology to your advantage, the more you will be amazed that you hadn't been using it all along. You may also recognize that there are some areas that you have been using it, and you can discover ways that you can tap into it even more and strengthen what is being used now. Applying the principles you learn about psychology will help you in a multitude of ways.

One could say that Walt Disney was a master at using psychology in growing his mega-company. He got to know the minds of his customers so intensely that he created a customer experience that is like no other. In fact, what he created, to please one's mind, is so successful that millions of people travel to Disney theme parks each year to experience it. You can only create something as huge as Disneyland or Disney World when you consider psychology and use the information you gain to your advantage, and much to the advantage of your customer.

When a business uses psychology correctly, it isn't just about helping their bottom line. It will do that, but it is so much more beyond just doing that. It's also about helping to create the best possible patient experience so that people want to keep coming back and they want to refer their friends and family. When you consider how your patients think, as well as others who you come into contact with, that information can go a long way toward helping to give your office a major boost.

Psychology is the understanding of personality traits of those around you, including your future patients, current patients, employees, referral sources, and others. It's understanding how people think and how things make them feel. There are a variety of ways you can use it to help create a great patient experience in your office. Psychology is quite literally the study of the human mind and its functions that affect behavior. Understanding psychology helps you better understand your patients, so you know more about their behavior, how they think, and the various things they may be feeling.

Practical Usage

For years, I have been beating up orthodontists I work with, saying "Listen, if you can't get patients to wear elastics or to wear an appliance or to brush their teeth, there are two ways to look at it." One is that you have crappy patients. If that's the case, then you have nobody to blame but yourself. You attracted those patients into your practice, so you have yourself to blame for them being there. The other option is that it's your fault. You didn't go a good enough job encouraging them, motivating them, and holding them accountable.

Owning the area of psychology involves getting better at patient cooperation, patient referrals, and building service value through understanding human nature. If you haven't read the book "The Social Animal," by Elliot Aronson,

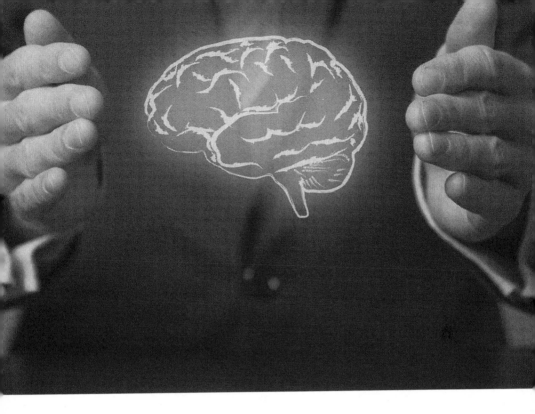

which most probably read in college, then I highly recommend checking it out. It's the definitive text that is in its 11th edition now. If you haven't read it, or it's been a long time, go back and read it. I guarantee it will help you.

It's not that our patients don't want to listen to you when you give them advice or ask them to do things for their treatment. They do. They want to do a good job and they want to have great teeth. The problem is that you haven't given them a good enough reason to do it yet. There's no motivation or accountability. You take two seconds to tell them to brush better, or wear their rubber bands, but that's not enough to motivate them to actually do those things, so the directive goes in one ear and out the other. There's a totally different and more effective way to do it, and that's where the idea of owning psychology comes into it. Maybe this is your area.

Maybe psychologically, you become the best orthodontist at helping patients get better results. What would doing that look like for your practice? Your success rate goes up, you have more happy people speaking your name out on the streets, more referrals come in, and the process continues, with your office excelling as it does. All these great benefits come because you owned the idea of understanding the human mind and using that information to create a better experience for both you and your patient.

In addition to determining how you can create a great experience for your patients, you can use the principles of psychology to do other things, too.

Some of them include, but are not limited to:

- Use it in your marketing to determine what appeals to people. What is it that makes people choose a particular orthodontist, respond to an ad, or finally pick up the phone for an appointment?

- Determine what facts you can use to get people to go forward with treatment. This will help raise your conversion rate. The people are coming in through the door because they usually need some kind of treatment. Learning more about how they think and what motivates them gives you tools to help motivate them more to make the commitment.

- Use psychology to make a better connection to your patients, referral sources, and employees. When you have a better understanding of basic psychology, you will often know why it is that people say what they say and do what they do. This can help with everything from your office synergy to helping to avert disasters.

- As mentioned earlier, you can use the information to help get people to be more motivated to adhere to their treatment. You will have a better understanding of their fears, challenges, and what roadblocks keep holding them back, and then help them learn to get over them.

- Apply the principles of psychology in your professional and private life. Using it in your private life will help strengthen your relationships, which leads to a happier you. When you are happy, that positive energy will transcend throughout your office.

- Using it to help determine what it is that motivates someone to make a referral. Then you can focus on strengthening that area, so you get more referrals.

- Psychology can even be used to get a more effective result out of your social media efforts. You can use it to determine what it is that people respond to, how they will react, how to use emotional triggers, and to better understand your audience and target market. If you take the time to learn more about your audience and target market, you will determine what inspires them, amuses them, and what motivates them to engage.

There are additional areas of psychology that you can use to help with your own business success. Consider something that most people think of as benign, such as the color they paint their walls in their practice or the color of the carpeting in the waiting area. While you may think that it has no impact, as long as it's clean and neat, those who know about psychology know otherwise.

In fact, color psychology is a real thing and one that can make a difference in your office. If you use color psychology to your advantage, you will be able to help change the way your patients feel. For example, the color of the walls can help influence how people feel. *Red is known for making people feel alive and alert, while green makes people feel calm and at ease, yellow makes people feel happy.* If you choose to own psychology, investigate color psychology and take a look at your office. You may decide that it's time to give it a facelift that will help to change the moods of those who walk through the doors.

Additionally, owning the area of psychology means having a basic understanding of the simple needs that every human has. Knowing these will help you be able to provide your patients with a better experience and one that is more personalized. Some of the basic needs that everyone has include being able to avoid pain, wanting variety, the need to feel important, being close with others, and being useful to other people. Everyone wants to feel listened to, understood, and cared about. This means treating each patient like family, rather than a dollar sign or another number closer to your quarterly goal. Armed with this knowledge, you can use it to help make a connection with your patients, help them overcome their fears, and to make them feel more comfortable.

Using Psychology Effectively

When you understand basic psychology, you can do a lot to make your office a better place. You can make it a great place, even better than any other place around. That's owning it, and it's completely possible through the use of psychology. You take what you learn, determine how you can use it to help your practice, and you roll with it, perfecting it as you go along.

One of the most important things you can do with using psychology is to create a better patient experience. Go through every step of the experience and see what needs to be improved and what is working. After watching many hours of secret shopper videos at orthodontic practices around the country, I can tell you that this is a huge issue. We've seen plenty of things on these videos that let us know that many orthodontists haven't given any thought at all to the patient experience. They only see the patient from their own point of view and often treat them that way.

Every patient who calls your office, has a consultation and receives treatment should feel like they had a great experience. They should always walk away from your office feeling like something good took place there, rather than walking away feeling bad, neglected, or unheard. If they leave your office with a positive feeling, then you and everyone in your office will have done their job right and will have furthered the mission of your practice. You can only become highly successful people if you love what you are doing and are excited to tell others about it and their experience there.

When using psychology, you want to focus on being positive. This should go without saying, but psychology itself is not synonymous with positivity. You can understand people and how they feel and act, but may be negative about it. Positivity is going to always create a better patient experience, so make keeping everything positive a high priority in your office. This doesn't mean that you will never encounter problems or unhappy patients. That is bound to happen. The most successful companies in the world still have a small percentage of people who are unhappy for whatever reason. Maybe they were in a bad mood, or someone in your office was. Maybe personalities didn't click, or perhaps there was a miscommunication so their expectations were off.

No matter what the reason is for the patient to be unhappy, or for the employee to be unhappy and possibly disgruntled, there is a positive and negative way to go about dealing with it. Whenever possible, and it's almost always possible, take the positive route. Take the high road that will leave your office looking better and help the unhappy person feel better about their experience. And always, always make things right if you know you have messed up somehow. Nobody likes to admit to mistakes, but when you own up to them you will gain a tremendous amount of respect from people.

When you go a step further to make it right, or as right as you possibly can, you will become an elite in their eyes. Admit when you're wrong. I've made millions of dollars and prevented countless lawsuits with two simple words, "I'm sorry."

Being able to help change the direction of something gone amiss is a part of psychology. Understanding psychology will help you pick up on behavioral cues, triggers and ways to help defuse situations. You can use it to help with issues on the phone, in the office and even through the messages you may receive on social media. Psychology gives you the background and tools to help you know how to effective communicate to get the conversation headed in a better direction.

Psychological Power

We've already discussed how you can use the power of understanding positive psychology to create a great patient experience. There are additional ways you can use it, too. These include using it in the areas of innovation and overcoming setbacks and challenges. Being in tune with how people feel and react to things will provide you with plenty of opportunity for coming up with new ideas. Innovation will become easier when you begin looking at things through the eyes, or mindset, of others.

Psychology can also be a major driving force in helping your business become a huge success, in part because you will understand the power of your own thoughts. Some people refer to it as positive thinking, while others call it the laws of attraction. But our thoughts go a long way toward determining how successful we are at something. It's the glass is half empty or half full scenario. If you know psychology, you realize how important having a positive mind can be, and what you can do to help to change your mood and become a happier person.

Every entrepreneur on the planet experiences some challenges and setbacks. Those who don't know how to handle those challenges, or who don't remain positive, will often be the ones who don't make it and end up closing their doors. Those who understand the power of their mind and psychology will usually find a way around it, through it, and over it. They will be the survivors who come out on top each and every time. Each of us is where we are today largely because of the decisions we have made all along, leading up to today. That's how powerful our minds are and how powerful they can be going forward. You just need to leverage that power to your advantage.

As a leader, you can use the power of psychology in numerous ways. Every effective leader has an understanding of psychology, because their job is to bring out the best in their team. You can only bring out the best in people if you understand how they think, feel, and what will make them have a positive experience. Focusing on psychology will help you be able to get your team in the right mindset, focusing on being positive, optimistic, happy, and resilient. It will give them the motivation to want to work together as a team, treat each patient with the best possible care, and provide the most amazing patient experience in the entire area.

The principles of psychology can help you get your foot in the door at referring dental offices, help you to be more persuasive, and understanding. One of the most important aspects to getting referrals, as previously mentioned, is building relationships with those who would make ideal referral sources. You can be more effective at relationship building when you employ the tool of understanding psychology.

Owning It

Psychology is a great area to own and one that will help propel your practice to the top. When you understand psychology, you will understand your patients, your referral sources, your employees, and everyone you come in contact with. You may not understand them completely, because even Freud was a bit wishy washy when it came to understanding the human mind, but you will understand them a whole lot better than every other practice in town.

Owning the area of psychology in your practice means using it for everything that you can think of, including when it comes to hiring, marketing, patient experience, interacting with others, and more. It gives you an edge, so that you have a better idea of how to keep the interaction positive and to help ensure that others get something out of the experience, too. It's not all about making sure you get the better end of the stick. When you give others a great experience and make them feel understood and cared about, they get a lot out of it, too. Psychology is a win-win situation when it comes to choosing an area to own. The more you know about how to deal with others, the better off the interaction will be.

What do you have to do to own the area of psychology? It doesn't require earning a degree in it, but you do need to take the time to learn about the basics. You can do that by reading The Social Animal by Elliot Aronson, in its twelfth edition at the time of this writing. Look up the most-commonly cited authors in the index. Ask your local librarian to pull those articles for you and highlight the common themes. Watch some movies and take an online class or at-home study course with The Great Courses. Get to one of my live events where we teach and practice these principles with you and your employees. Do these things, and you'll be an expert in psychology compared to every other orthodontist.

There's a really good chance that no other orthodontist in your area has excelled in the area of psychology. If you choose this area you will be a one-of-a-kind orthodontist probably within at least a 100-mile radius. That's a great thing and something to consider. Having patients leave your practice feeling understood, appreciated and positive will go a long way toward helping your practice grow.

Besides, the field of psychology is an interesting one. Some estimate that we will encounter around 80,000 people in our lifetime. Imagine how much better our interactions will be both in the office and outside it if we have a better understanding of basic human psychology. It's a great area to choose to own because it can essentially benefit you in every area of your life and then some.

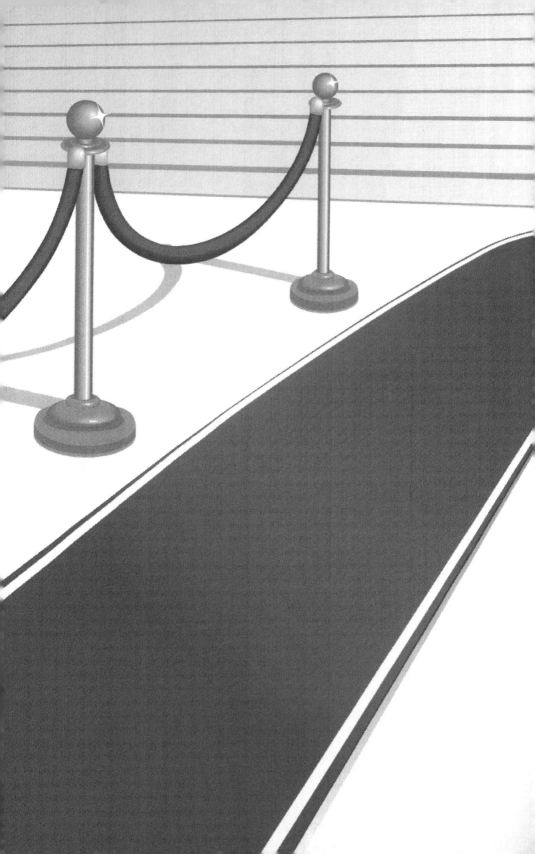

CHAPTER NINE
HOSPITALITY

*"Try not to become a man of success.
Rather become a man of value."- Albert Einstein*

Value is something that your office provides to every patient. Granted, how much value you are providing is dependent upon the type of service and patient experience that you are offering. If people visit your office and walk out feeling like they have had a great experience, then you are providing a lot of value. On the other hand, if they walk out feeling something was lacking, that you didn't live up to expectations, or even worse, then you are not providing much value at all.

Hospitality is the cornerstone of value in any industry. Typically speaking, people often think of the hotel and resort industry when they think of the word hospitality. However, it's a term that can be used across the board in business. It's the treatment of people, including being generous and friendly. The resort industry may be synonymous with the word, simply because when we check into a place we want all of our needs met and we want to be treated with kindness and for those working there to be friendly. Whether we need extra pillows or we forgot our toothbrush, we turn to the resort staff for assistance, and their commitment to hospitality provides us with these things, served up with a smile.

We can and should do the same in our offices. *Nailing hospitality means that you are going to be committed to the idea of going above and beyond for every one of your patients.* It's about treating them with kindness, generosity, and giving them an awesome patient experience, so that they get a lot of value out of their visit. In today's fast-paced world, hospitality is often an area that is sorely lacking. People are busy, distracted, and focused on what's next, instead of what's right in front of them. We can do better than that, and if you choose to own the area of hospitality you will.

Better Than the Rest

Service, customer service, hospitality – what do you do consistently, over and over again, better than your competitors? This is such an important area that if you choose to own it, you have to change the way you and your employees look at the entire process. In fact, we did in our office. We think of it as a show, similar to the mindset at Disney, and our office is the stage. Before each employee goes on stage, they have to remember that they are a part of a show. Their job is to provide the best possible patient experience, despite what may be going on in their life.

I get it, and so do your patients, that people have issues going on in their life. Everyone does. We know that your dog is sick, or you wrecked your car last week, or that you've just had a really bad day. We get it, because we have all been there. But what happens if you, or your employees, take the frustrations and attitudes that come with these things and let them hang around while taking care of patients? What happens is that they get a poor experience. If your employees are having a bad week or something is going on in their lives, they shouldn't project that onto the patients. If they do, the entire patient experience will suffer.

You and your patients need to perform and put on the best show, just like they do at Disney. Don't you think that the people who work at Disney also have a list of issues they are dealing with in their private lives? They probably hit major traffic heading into work, because it's always backed up in those areas, and they may have a dozen other things go on. But they don't step into being a part of the show and let their angst or attitude come through to the guest. The guest watches their show and sees a great performance every time.

In our office, we know that we have a show to perform. These patients are only here for 30 minutes, every 8 or 12 weeks. In all honesty, they don't really care that your car is broken down, your dog is sick, or that you have had a bad day. Frankly, they just want to get what they are paying for as quickly as possible, so they can get on with their day. And they want to get that with people who

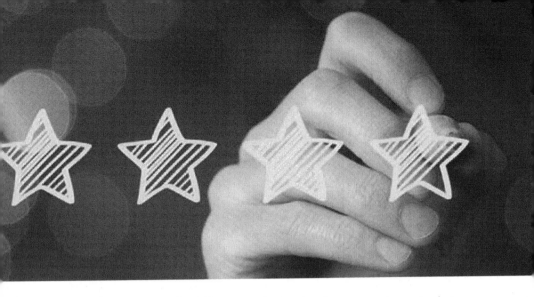

are smiling and being friendly, not with people who are caught up in their own world of issues and bringing everyone else down around them.

I'm not trying to sound mean here, but I've watched plenty of secret shopper videos that back up what I'm saying. I see patients walk into an office and get subpar treatment because the employee didn't have a good lunch, got an unhappy text from their spouse, or is struggling with a private issue. Showing those things to your patients is not the time or place. Those things have no place in the show that is your patient experience. Maybe they get that unhappy text, but then they realize they are in a show at the moment, and they realize they need to get back immediately to playing the part.

Your patients want their problems solved, and they want to go home. That's the bottom line. They don't want to sit around your office any longer than they have to, no matter how nice and comfortable you may make it. They want certain things from us, and they are entitled to them. They are not paying for drama, to listen to sob stories, or to get treated in a subpar manner because your employee is having a bad day. We can and should always do better than that. Disney never suffers or is subpar because employees aren't having an amazing day, and the same should go for our office.

Service Steps

In our office, we have defined service steps. We know exactly how we want our patient experience to be, so we have taken the steps to make it happen. We've defined it and created the set of steps that everyone in the office can follow to make it happen. Now, keep in mind that these are only the steps. They are not the attitude with which each step is completed. The attitude is something that has to be covered, so that employees realize they are part of the show that will go on at your office. *Merely going through the steps you set up is only half of the equation. The steps need to be done by employees who remember why they are there, which is to provide amazing service to every patient.*

Our service steps are defined by the acronym SMILE. We say hello and greet the patient by name. We do what we can to make them feel at home. We avoid saying things like "We'll be right with you." You wouldn't say that to a guest in your home, and you should be treating your patients with the same level of respect. If you were to have a party tonight or were hosting a holiday party at your home, you wouldn't bring people into your living room and say something like "I'll be right with you. Sit over there. Here's a clipboard, fill out this paperwork." Not at all. You would say something more like "Oh, you must be Billy. Who did you bring with you? We've been waiting for you. You're going to meet with Ashley. You are going to love her, she's great. Come on back. Let me show you where you are going. Here's our office, let me give you a tour."

The second service step is M, for Make them feel at home. If someone came to visit your home, you would bring the person in and make them feel comfortable and at home right away. You'd want to make them feel like they had come to the right place and that they were wanted there. How you would treat the people who come to your home for a party is the same manner that you should use to greet and treat people in your office. Your office is essentially an extension of your home. You are welcoming these patients into your second home and into your life, so let's do it with some authenticity, genuine interest, and with great hospitality.

The third service step in our practice is I, for Invite. We invite them to share. We make a plan for the next step, by asking something like "Tell us what brought you in today" or "How have you been since our last visit?" We want to move forward on the patient's terms, so we're always inviting them to share. People will tell you exactly what they want from you if you invite them to do so. So we're constantly asking the patient to share "What's next?" in our journey together.

Then we listen. The fourth service step is L, for Listen. We let people tell us exactly what they want and then we give it to them. Listening to your patients is such an important thing that many doctors overlook. People will tell you what the problem is and what they want, but often times, doctors are not tuned into listening to the patient. A study at the Mayo Clinic found that it only takes 16 seconds, on average, for a doctor to interrupt a patient after asking him or her a question.

The final service step is E, for End with a Fond Farewell. At Zingerman's Deli, one of my favorite companies from Ann Arbor, Michigan, they call it their 10/4 rule. Within 10 feet of any customer, they acknowledge who's in front of them. They look up and smile. Within four feet they use an actual greeting. "Hello, how are you? Good morning." They don't allow employees to avoid eye contact and interaction with customers. They actively engage at 10 feet and 4 feet. Think about how many companies break the 10/4 rule. Zingerman's Deli refuses to avoid their customers. Pretty smart for a place that serves sandwiches. You're serving something much more expensive and frightening to consumers than pastrami on rye. Do you take your service steps as seriously as most delis? I hope so.

At our practice, we eat, live and breathe the Five Service Steps. We smile and we greet the patient by name. We make them feel at home. We invite them to share and we listen. Then we always end with a fond farewell, and we invite them to come back. This is something we do each and every time, it is non-negotiable. It's embedded into our culture and subconscious.

Improving Your Show

When you see a show in action, it may look flawless to you. The people in the show make it look easy, like it's something they have always done. What you don't see is the significant amount of time and effort invested in order to define and design the show. Who plays each part and how the show should unfold; the pace and timing of every muscle movement – that's exactly what you need to do with the patient experience and their complete lifecycle within your practice.

Regardless of how your hospitality has been up to this point, you can absolutely become better at it and you can own this area in your market. A great book

(S) SAY hello and greet every guest by name.

The most important word in the world to any person is their first name. Use it. Leverage it to build trust and relationships then mine those relationships for the mutual benefit of both parties.

(M) MAKE them feel at home.

Offer a beverage, take their coat, treat them as a guest in your home. You wouldn't tell your house guest to take a seat and you'll be "right with them" would you? No. Instead, you would go out of your way to make them feel at home. Do the same with every patient interaction.

(I) INVITE them to share and make a plan for the next step.

How have they been, what brings them in today, how can you help? Make it a point to invite your patients to share with you exactly where they are in the process of transforming their smile: confused, nervous, overwhelmed, ready to get started, still have lots of questions, etc. Patients will tell you exactly what they want from you, if you'll just invite them to share.

(L) LISTEN for and resolve questions or special requests.

Patients are their parents have unexpressed wishes or desires - things that are important to them but they might not voice. If you listen for the things that are important to the patient and parent, you can get to the heart of the matter quickly.

(E) END with a fond farewell and an invitation to return.

The last thing people remember about your practice is the send off or farewell. You cannot skimp on this area. A patient or parent in your practie might only see you for 30 minutes every 8-12 weeks. Your interaction during that time and particularly at the end of the appointment needs to be special. Don't let your patient leave without a reason to come back and share something.

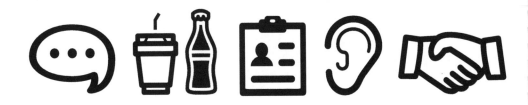

to read on this topic is called "Small Data: The Tiny Clues That Uncover Huge Trends." Written by a man who was hired by leading brands around the world to find out the little pieces of data that make their customers tick, the information is invaluable. I've read a lot of books. A lot. So I don't typically get really excited about most books, but this one by Martin Lindstrom is brilliant.

The author of the book actually goes and lives, with permission, with the people who he is gathering data about for these companies. He kind of moves in with the people, eats all meals with them, is allowed to go through their drawers, is allowed to go through their phones and Twitter accounts, and even see what type of emojis people use. Keep in mind that he's hired by big companies like IBM and Lego. He gets million-dollar contracts. Lego's one of his biggest clients that hired him to figure out how to turn the company around years ago.

The information he gathers and shares is eye-opening and can be used by any type of business in order to understand people better and create a better patient experience. I have seen a lot of these data issues myself through watching thousands of hours of secret shopper videos. The data is there for those watching and paying attention. The point here is that the small things matter. The little bits of data about your patients matter. This book by Martin Lindstrom made me realize just how much the little things matter. If you are going to own the area of hospitality, you have to go searching for the little bits of data. You have to get out the magnifying glass and go searching, because all of that information about your patients is going to make a huge difference. Use that information to know more about your patients and create the best patient experience in your market.

Uncovering Little Things

The little things matter more than we realize, which is something that is often overlooked, at least until someone puts it in front of us and makes us realize it. When we put the data under a magnifying glass and gain a better picture of who our patients are and what makes them tick, we will be able to better reach them, work with them, and create an experience that will exceed their expectations. While you can't do as this author did by going to essentially move in with your patients, you can do a lot of digging and pay attention, so that you can build your own little book of data about them.

There is a lot you can discover that needs to be worked on when you start looking at the little stuff. One of those things is the average wait time that a patient experiences, starting from the moment their hand touches the door to walk in. Not just how long they sit in the reception area, but the entire time they are at your office. Just because they are sitting and waiting in a room doesn't mean their time is no longer passing them by, because it is. Every minute they sit in a room just waiting for something to happen counts, and it counts more than you may realize.

We have measured thousands of hours of secret shopper video to assess the data. What we have found is that from the time the patient puts their hand on the door until something meaningful takes place, such as taking photos or radiographs or actually talking about what brought them in, the time elapsed is about 21 minutes. This is an average across the board on videos we have watched. Sure, there are some that are as little as three minutes, and others that wait as long as an hour before something meaningful takes place, but 21 minutes is the average. These are not dumb doctors, mind you. Our average orthodontic client has over $2.5 million in annual revenue. They are well above the national average. So why is this happening?

Well, for a lot of the reasons mentioned earlier, it's because employees don't see themselves as playing a role in the show. They see themselves as performing a job, and they let everything else that's going on in their lives get in the way. The job they feel they are performing is, "I've got enough patients. I've got more patients than I can deal with, and right now I really just want to get to lunch on time. So here's some paperwork, go fill this out." That's 21 minutes wasted from the time they put their hand on the front door until the time something meaningful happens.

This is absolutely insane. This is no way to provide good hospitality and it's certainly not providing people with a great patient experience. One thing that we should all keep in mind is that your patient's time is every bit as valuable as your own time. We wouldn't be pleased with our patients all showing up 21 minutes late for their appointments, so we should give them the same respect in return. If their appointment is at 2:00, then every effort should be made to have something meaningful taking place at 2:00. That's treating them how we would want to be treated.

In our office, I know that six minutes is all I need in the new patient room if everything else is performed correctly. The paperwork is done and even if they haven't completed it ahead of time, give me six minutes with the patient and I can comfortably get to the heart of the matter and come to an agreement on the next steps we're going to take together.

This is so different than their experience at other doctor's offices that patients and parents often say "I wish other doctors ran their offices like this place. We didn't have to wait at all." The six minutes is all I really need to listen to the patient or parent and determine if braces are going to be necessary or not, if clear aligners are a better option or not and whether or not we are going to do it now or wait until later. Parents really want to know if our office is the right place to trust with their child's smile. Give me six minutes and all of this will be determined and agreed upon. So why do most orthodontists spend 60 minutes for new patient exams?

Orthodontists schedule an hour for new patients because 21 minutes of the appointment is completely wasted. But if you don't go looking for the clues and little pieces of data, you don't realize that. If you are not watching secret shopper videos, you never see all the wasted time in action and realize what's going on. You will never know, because you don't even realize the new patient is in the office until your team says "Dr. Smith, there's a new patient ready in exam room one." You have no idea you've wasted 21 minutes of this person's time and as a profession, we can do better.

Our practices put an end to this insanity the minute we realized that's what was going on. Nobody wants 21 minutes of their life wasted in our office, just waiting for something to happen. We never want our patient experience to include 21 minutes of wasted idle time in our office. Either find a way to make meaningful use of those 21 minutes, narrow your appointments down or do both. Figure this out before your next new patient comes to your office and has their time wasted. I can assure you that most of you are wasting way too much time in the new patient room, but if you own the area of hospitality and start watching secret shopper video, that problem will be quickly solved once and for all.

Owning It

You can see now that there are ways that you can improve your hospitality. Start by evaluating your patient experience and looking for the little things that can be improved. You want to be known for providing the most amazing patient experience in your market. You do that by not wasting the patient's time, by being a great listener, by anticipating what they will need and when they will need it and by respecting them.

When you treat every patient who comes through your doors like a superstar, you will own the area of hospitality. Make every person feel like a high roller when they walk through your door. When their hand opens the door your team goes into action, putting on the show that is going to make that patient feel special, welcomed, appreciated, and well cared-for. Patients should be treated like gold, because in essence, that's exactly what they are. Without them, you wouldn't have a practice.

This isn't to say that every patient who walks through your doors is going to be a great patient or that they are never wrong. You will have isolated cases that you need to deal with individually, but they are going to be few and far between, and they should never be representative of the entire experience. When isolated issues happen, always strive to find a solution to the best of your ability. Go out of your way to make things right. How people behave toward your office is a reflection of them, but how you and your employees respond is a reflection of you. Make sure that response sends the reflection of your office that you want it to and never change your patient experience for a few outliers. Deal with outliers individually but keeping running your show.

Owning Hospitality

I can tell you with absolute certainty that the area of hospitality is not one that most orthodontists own. 88% of companies think they provide great customer service but only 8% actually do. This presents a tremendous opportunity for those willing to take it seriously. Owning it means you will become the director in the show and ensure that everyone plays their part, so that the patients have a great experience every time they enter your office. It's a powerful area to own that will grow your referrals help you deliver more value to your patients than any other doctor in your market.

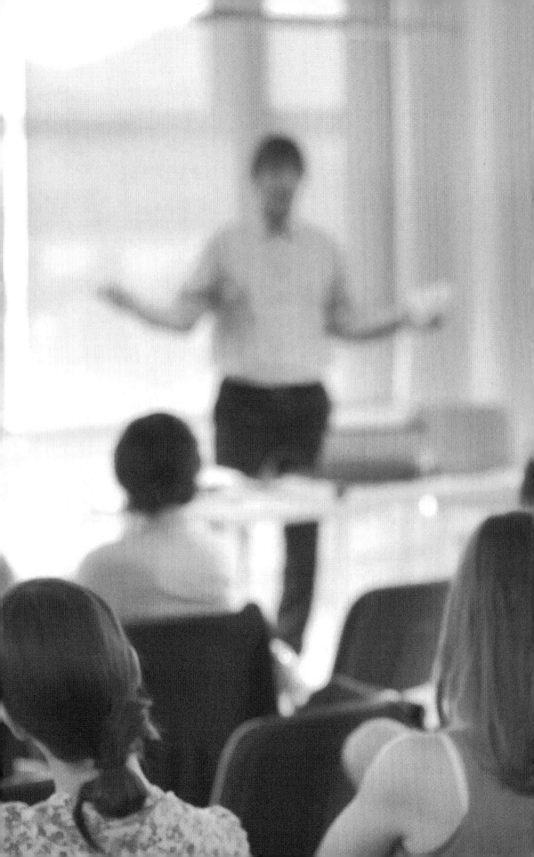

CHAPTER TEN
LIVE EVENTS

"Whatever the mind can conceive and believe, the mind can achieve." - Napoleon Hill

When is the last time your office put on an event, or took part in one that someone else was having? There's a good chance that you either don't know the answer to that question or you haven't considered the power of live events. Live events are something that tend to go under the radar for most orthodontists, yet they can be an incredible tool for helping to build your relationships, increasing referrals and keeping people talking about your office.

If you haven't been doing live events, now may just be the ideal time to give it some serious consideration. Choosing to own the area of live events will create wonderful opportunities for your office. It's an area that reaches beyond what most doctors would even consider, leaving you a lot of room for standing out, getting noticed, and keeping in contact with a much larger audience. These are things that will all benefit your office in numerous ways, so they're always worth considering.

Why Events Rule
Consulting with orthodontists around the world, I know that most have never been involved in doing live events. Most have no idea why they would do it, how to go about it and whether or not it's even worth the investment of their time and money. Well, I'm here to offer a resounding yes, that it is well worth the time and money invested, and that owning the area of live events can provide huge growth for your practice.

At our office, I like to think of us as being in the event business. We do a wide variety of events, including a lot of continuing education events. Every year, we bring in lots of doctors and hygienists. We schedule lunch and learn events, where attendees get a special topic presented to them, along with a free catered lunch. I'm not talking about going from office to office, talking about orthodontics to individual dental offices. I did that and it was exhausting. It's much more efficient to invite a local expert like a CPA or financial planner to speak at an event for a large group doctors at one time.

Your accountant can speak to the group about tax strategies or another topic that would be interesting enough to fill the room. Those in attendance are all potential referral sources, mind you. Hold an event offering tax strategies and you will probably get at least 100 doctors to attend the event. They listen to the presentation and have some great food. Meanwhile, you just connected with over 100 doctors in your area. You don't need to set up 100 different lunches or go to 100 different offices. All you need to do is walk around and talk to everyone at a larger event. That's where the networking takes place and you begin to build or strengthen relationships.

Today, we do a lot of this type of networking, and I'm happy to say that we do it a lot smarter than we used to. We learned along the way what the best ways were for identifying who should attend, what types of events will draw a crowd, how to manage them and the best way for me to connect with those who show up. You learn those things along the way if you are paying attention to what's going on. The more of these live events that you do, the better you become at them. You will become more efficient at their timing, planning, and executing, helping your office to get an even better return on investment.

Like any of the areas presented in this book, the one that you choose to own will be one that you feel comfortable with and you believe you will be able to master. Doing live events may not be the right one to own if you are someone who despises events or crowds. But if it you like the idea of networking with a lot of people and simplifying the process to do it, then by all means this may be the area that is right for your office. Owning live events means you are going to be better than any other office in your area when it comes to holding events that will help facilitate networking, as well as for having fun and building relationships.

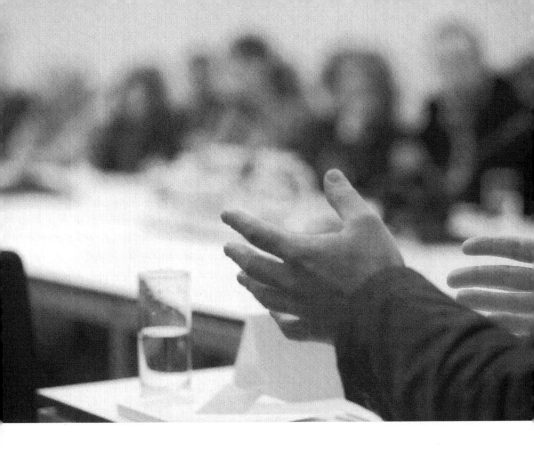

The cornerstone of any orthodontic practice is a steady stream of referrals. The most effective way to have a strong referral system is to build the relationships that will lead to them. This is a big step in the right direction for networking and building those relationships. Having live events may seem like a monumental task right now, but that's probably just because you are not used to having them. Get a few of them under your belt and you will realize how easy, and most importantly how effective, they can be.

Networking is the major reason to engage in live events and to consider owning the area. However, it's not the only benefit that your practice will get from having live events. You will also benefit because you will be positioning yourself as an expert in your field, as someone who others in the area turn to and look up to when they need orthodontic information. You will also benefit from generating awareness of your office and helping to build your brand name and image. This will give you a chance to interact with people outside your office, and will help you be able to expand your reach.

Another major benefit to having events is that you will give people a chance to come face to face with you. In today's world, we have massive amounts of things that are done through digital communication. You may interact with people through email and online that you never see in person. The live events will bring people together, which is where real connections take place. You strengthen relationships by having face-to-face contact. Think I'm wrong? Try raising your kids via Skype or instant message. Real relationships are built in the flesh and based on trust. Doctors are not going to enthusiastically or exclusively refer to you unless they trust you and have a strong relationship with you. Live events are critical to achieving these goals.

Events are also a great way to stand out as being a part of your community. As an orthodontist, you want people to see your office as a proud member and supporter of your community. Live events can give you that edge and show that you care about and enrich your local community. Events give people a chance to meet up with like-minded individuals. Depending on the types of events you have, they may also help your employees become more comfortable and masterful in their positions. They can showcase their own networking skills and as long as they are playing their part right in the show, they will help make your office look great.

What happens when people attend an event? What happens when you attend one? Chances are, some of the people who attend your events will end up checking in online to say they are there, and then talking about it later with others. The word of mouth mentions are worth a lot, as the events will get people talking and put your office name out there. That's all brand exposure and can end up benefiting your office. Take photos and encourage your attendees to share online with their friends and colleagues.

Types of Events

One of the great things about owning the area of live events is that you are only limited to your own imagination. The sky is the limit when it comes to the types of events you can engage in. Of course, you want to ensure they make sense for your practice to engage in, but there's plenty of room for ingenuity here. The variety of events that exist will offer different ways to network with professionals in your area, help build relationships with current and past patients, and get your office mingling with and being a part of the community. Here are some of the types of events, just to give you an idea of what's out there, but you are not bound by these alone:

Learning Events. These are the types of events that are focused on providing information. It may be information that you are offering, such as an orthodontic topic, or on something that will be useful to those you invite, such as the accountant speaking to local doctors about taxes. Learning events will get people interested because there's something they can get out of them that they may be able to use right away in their own practice. Learning events can take place in person or you can even have webinars. Those taking place in person can be held at your office if you have the space, or you can affordably rent a conference room at a local hotel or restaurant if you expect a large turnout.

Learning and educational events give you the ability to position yourself as an expert on the topic, and bring people in for networking. You want to attend those events even if you are not the one who will be speaking. They are a great opportunity to speak with everyone who attends and begin laying the foundation for a relationship. Everyone who attends needs to get some value out of it, so avoid having fluff. The last thing you want to do is waste people's time, because if they feel it was a waste of time they are not likely to attend another event in the future.

Lunch and learn events, or business breakfast events, don't have to be held every month in order for you to get a lot of mileage out of them. You can hold one every quarter or a couple of times per year, and if they are impactful, meaning people leave there having spent their time wisely, then your office will gain from it.

Having webinars is another way to have live events, but they don't call for you to plan an in-person event. I've had many of these, and they help you to reach a larger audience, but you don't have the personal connection that you would have at a face-to-face event. They won't be right for every situation, but the option for them is there if you can find a way for them to reach your target audience.

While we have mainly been touching on the idea of having educational events for the doctors in your area, there are others you can have them for as well. Consider all of the people who can benefit from the information, and in return may be a good referral source for your office. Those are all potential event participants. These include hygienists, school nurses, pediatricians and patients. Each of these people have something you can offer them, and by building a relationship with them you will get referrals in return. Just be sure that your event is tailored to the right audience and that they walk away feeling it was worth their time.

Educational events can also be held for the public, such as holding an "Everything you wanted to know about braces" event. The audience here would be parents and teens who are considering braces. Along with a talk format, you can offer a questions and answers segment, so that people can have their individual questions answered.

Just for Fun. At least it will look like the events are just for fun, but you and I both realize that there is another reason for them as well. Holding fun live events is a great way to connect with the community, network, and showcase your personality. I've said it before and I'll say it again: The last thing you can be is boring. Nobody talks about boring, but when you are in the office all of the time it's not always easy to let a more relaxed side of you shine through. When you have some events that are fun, you can be there showing people a different side of you. At fun events, you should always walk around to mingle with the attendees, allowing them to see you having fun and being relaxed. That gives them a chance to see your personality, which will also help to build trust and further your relationship building.

Just for fun events can be a great way to honor your VIPs. You should always know where your referrals come from. It's always surprising to me that many orthodontists have no idea, or very little idea, as to where their referrals come from. If you don't know where they are coming from it's difficult to tap that resource and get even more of them. By knowing where your referrals are coming from you can always keep tabs on your VIPs. Those are the people who continuously send you new patients. They send you good patients, and yes there are is a difference between good and bad patients. Your list of VIPs is a potential gold mine. That list should be coveted and the people on it should be treated with special attention and care. Let them know how much you appreciate them and you will absolutely continue to get even more referrals from this group of people.

Holding VIP events for those who are sending you a lot of referrals just makes good sense. We've held such events and we see the impact that it has, so we know that it works. VIP events should focus on making those attending feel, well, like very important people. They should have fun, be given some gifts, and be treated to a great time. You can have a VIP night once or twice a year, where you invite everyone on your VIP list. Give them all great gifts, food, fun times, and walk around and mingle with them all. You will be giving them a lot to talk about, they will love that you show your appreciation for them, and you will get more referrals as a result.

Everyone wants to be appreciated and feel important. Very few doctors will take the time to do this for their VIPs. Most doctors haven't even identified their VIPs and have no idea how many referrals they've sent in the last year. This presents a tremendous opportunity for you in your market.

When you have events where it makes sense to do so, considering setting up a photo booth or selfie station. It was estimated that in 2016, 1 billion selfies were taken per day. That's incredible amount, showing just how much people like to take selfies. Why should you care? Think about what people do when they take a selfie. Most of the time, they will share it on one or more of their social media platforms. When they do so, they are bound to do a check-in at your office, or to say they are at your VIP party. Each time that happens, it is a plug for your practice. Also, make the gifts that you give out at these events so great that people feel they have to take pictures of it and share it on their social media outlets. Again, your practice is associated with it all, helping to offer an implied trust and referral to your office. They are essentially endorsing you, without having to come out and say that in their post.

At your fun live events, you can further maximize your image branding by having a professional photographer document the activities. People online can see all the fun taking place, even if they were unable to attend. You can use the photos and videos in YouTube and Facebook posts to get more mileage out of them, showing people the fun your office engages in, and how your VIPs are treated. If those watching see how great the VIPs are treated, there's a good chance that some of them will want to make their way onto that list. That equals more referrals for you.

Your fun events shouldn't be limited to the VIP crowd, however. You certainly want to have some of them each year, but you also want to have some fun events for the community and your patients. In the summer time, for example, we have shown outdoor movies so that people can come enjoy a free movie under the stars, complete with snacks and prize giveaways. This type of event gives you a chance to mingle with people, helping to build relationships, shows you have a fun office, and helps to create a bond with your community.

Other People's Events. Take one look around your community and you are bound to find a plethora of live events taking place. Some of these may make sense for you to be a part of, even if it's setting up a booth in a community health fair. You will need to evaluate each of them to determine which ones make sense for your office to take part in. From sponsoring a 5K run to teaming up with the elementary schools to be a business partner at their on-campus events, there are a variety of ways to get involved in someone else's events. One of the advantages of doing this is that you don't have to plan the event and you have minimal expense and time involved. Typically, you would just show up and either speak, set up a table, or be involved as a sponsor. Some of these you also don't necessarily have to be there at, but you can have someone from your team there to represent your office.

One thing you don't want to forget if you go this route is marketing. The events you have should be served up with a side of marketing. Events should be reported to the media, promoted online, and even afterward there should be pictures posted online. You want to cover your bases here to make sure the community knows about the events and that you showcase how great they were after the fact.

Owning It

Owning the area of live events can be a fun endeavor. Perhaps you are someone who loves to mingle, network, and you are an extrovert. If so, then this is certainly an area for you to consider owning. If you are going to own it, then you want to excel in being a part of live events. You have to put on better events than any other doctors in your area, the kind that get people talking. You want people to discuss how your office puts on great events and how fun and/or educational they are.

Don't fear not having the time to plan all of the events and every detail about them. This is a job that someone in your office can easily manage. Choose the person who you know will shine in this area, and make it their project. While you will play a role in determining what type of event you will have and you will be there to mingle and network, that person can take care of all of the details and get everything set up for you.

Many people love live events. They bring people together, giving you a chance to relax and mingle with others. It gives people a chance to save time and be able to network with colleagues at the same time. And when done right, they can become a great source of boosting your referrals. Hosting and taking part in great events puts you out there in the community, gets your office noticed, and helps position you in a way you want to be noticed.

You are limited only to your imagination when it comes to choosing the events you want to take part in. Think big and think fun, different, and helpful. Give people a chance to have fun and learn something in your name. Good things will happen when you own the area of live events, both for your office and referral strategies, as well as for your standing in the community.

"One customer, well taken care of, could be more valuable than $10,000 worth of advertising." - Jim Rohn

---

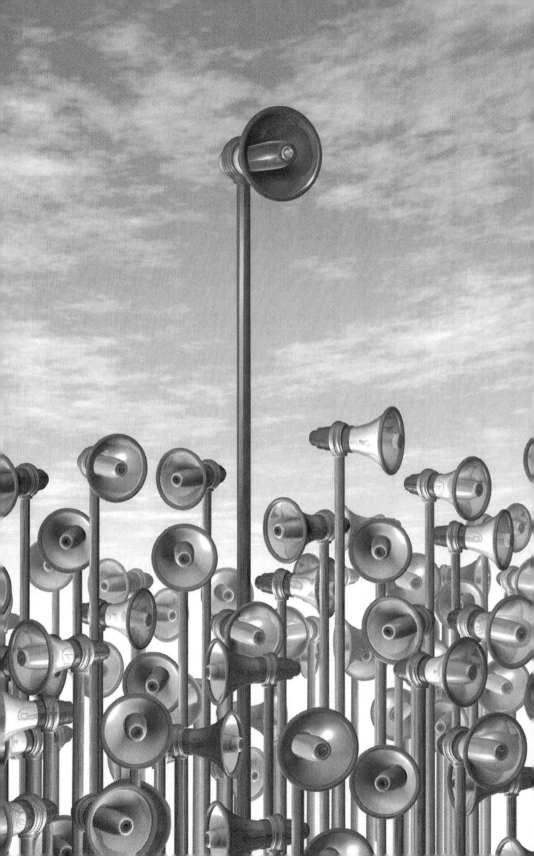

CHAPTER ELEVEN
PUBLIC RELATIONS

"Publicity, publicity, publicity is the greatest moral factor and force in our public life." - Joseph Pulitzer

When you think about how much your office interacts with the greater public, you can see that the idea of having a good relationship with them is a great idea. The public, after all, is the people we want to come in for appointments, but it is also made up of those in the community, including people we want to network with, reporters who can write stories on what we do, and others who can either help share about our favorable image or send referrals our way.

Maintaining a positive relationship with everyone outside your office doors is a wise thing to do. Owning this area is one that is not only wise, but will bring you a great deal of benefits in return. Just imagine having a great relationship with everyone in the community outside your office. That includes local dentists, schools, pediatricians, health reporters, and so on. What would that do for your office and reputation? Well, in fact, I can tell you without a doubt that it would do a lot for your office, including for your reputation, expertise status and referrals.

The term "public relations" is one that often confuses people, because they are not quite sure what it entails. It's also one that scares people a little bit. That again is largely because they don't understand what it is and how they would go about managing it. Public relations is nothing to run from. In fact, it can be an important tool for your practice when used right. It can help keep you in the good graces of many, get you media attention when you need it most and can help strengthen your brand image.

Even if you don't choose to own the area of public relations, your office will greatly benefit from learning more about what it is, how to use it to your advantage and in putting some of it into practice. In fact, as you learn more about what public relations really is, there is a good chance you will wonder how you have been getting by so long without it. There are simple ways to use it that will have a big payoff, so it should become a part of every practice's management plans.

Owning the area of public relations means that you are going to do it better than any other orthodontist in your area. You are going to master the skills, leverage the power, and use it to help carve your personal path to success. I've seen how powerful using public relations can be, so I know this is an area that you will want to give serious consideration. With proper management, you can have a lot of control and influence over how the public views your office and brand.

Public Relations Defined

If you were to ask half a dozen people what public relations is, you would be lucky to find one who actually had a correct answer. The truth of the matter is that most people don't know what it is and many who do have a difficult time explaining it. Dig a little deeper and you will get plenty of definitions to help shed some light on the subject. The Public Relations Society of America defines it as a strategic communication process that builds mutually beneficial relationships between organizations and their people.

Recall that one of the absolute most important things you can do for your referral system strategy is to build good relationships with people. That's with referring dentists, hygienists, school nurses, pediatricians, current patients, and so on. You get the idea, which is that when you build good relationships with the public you will help to elevate your practice. People will want to refer you, because they know you and trust you. When it comes down to it, then, public relations is nothing more than the strategy that is used to help build and strengthen those relationships. How could that be anything but a positive for any business out there?

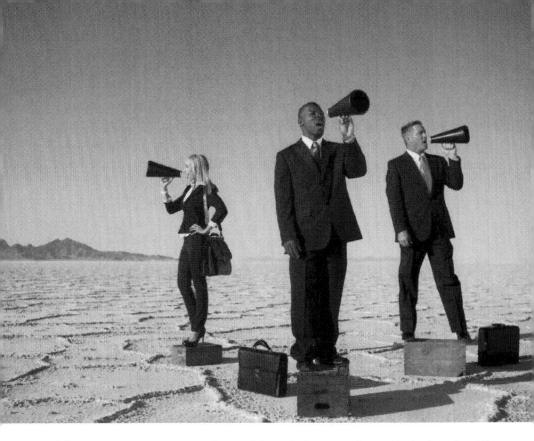

There are numerous ways that public relations can be used, and each will influence what you get back in return. There is the public relations that you can use to network with other professional contacts, that which helps keep you on the radar of the local health reporter, and that which helps assure that the community at large holds a favorable opinion of your services. Owning public relations means you will tap into each of the areas, so you can get the benefits that will come from every avenue you energetically explore.

There's a concept that I call "Keeping people in orbit around you." How do you keep people in orbit around you? I'm referring to your vendors, employees, community leaders, religious leaders, coaches, even the school board and PTA president. All of those people and what it entails to keep in contact with each of those people. Make no mistake, keeping each of these people, and many others in your community, in your orbit is very important. That's the essence of public relations.

If you are like most people, you probably don't have a list of 100 people you touch base with at least a couple of times per year. In a sense, that's your public relations list. It's the list of 100 people who you want to make sure you maintain a connection with, or keep them in your orbit. These are the people you should send a handwritten card to, a birthday gift, maybe an encouraging note, a book you think they would like, maybe a cute trinket you find on vacation. It's about sending them something once or twice per year to show that you are thinking of them and keeping them in your orbit.

Do you know someone that you used to keep in touch with, who used to inspire you or help your practice or in your personal life, who you fell out of contact with? Perhaps it was your bicycling buddy, yoga pal, or first Tuesday of the month lunch bunch crowd. Perhaps you have had a friend or colleague who you've let fall out of your orbit. How many times have you blamed the other person for this happening? You say things like, "Well, he never calls." But you don't stop to realize that the street goes both ways. You have a phone, too.

You get the idea. If you want to keep people in your orbit, you can't just hope that you will remember and keep on keeping on. You need a more systematic approach to maintaining those relationships, which is where public relations comes into play.

If you want to have those people come back into your orbit, you must give them a reason to come back around. I've got news for you. If the sun wasn't heating this planet, our orbit around it would be pointless. We would be one big ice ball. There's a reason our orbit around the sun is important. So what reasons are you giving people to stay in touch with you? Too many of us blame the other person. A dentist stops referring patients to us and it's easy to blame the dentist. When was the last time you got real and asked yourself why they stopped referring? What where you doing to maintain that relationship and keep that dentist in your orbit in the first place?

You can't just put relationships on autopilot and assume all those people will remain in orbit around you. Yes, maintaining those relationships will take some time, but it will be well worth the investment, and you can also get the assistance of someone in your office to help with this. You bring back a trinket from a vacation that you think is perfect for someone on your list, and you can always have your employee send it to them.

Our office is in Kansas City so I send a lot of barbecue to people throughout the world. I know people within my orbit appreciate the surprise of a tasty barbecue package being delivered to their office, and so I make it a point do send these to people throughout the year. I don't get any bonus points in this orbit example if I merely think about sending these people some barbecue. Our thoughts and actions are two different things. We can think about people in our orbit often, but unless we take some sort of action there will be no connection. They don't know you are thinking about them. You have to reach out at least twice a year to connect and show them somehow that you are thinking of them. I only get points for actually sending the barbecue, and you will only get points for the things you do. It's the action that is going to count and keep people in your orbit, not merely thoughts about what you would like to do.

Different Forms

As mentioned, there are various directions you can take with maintaining your public relations. You may know someone who hires a PR firm that handles their public relations. In essence, that firm is taking care of one aspect of managing their public relations, but certainly not all of it. What PR firms are great at doing is getting you media exposure, image branding, and helping to keep your media contacts within your orbit. But they don't focus on much more beyond that. If they did, you would be working for them. It's your practice. You can get help with this area but you must own PR.

Many people confuse this form of public relations with advertising. There's a big difference, though. With advertising, you are paying for ads and you are saying something about your practice. With public relations, such as when a PR firm works on your behalf, they work on getting others to showcase your office and say good things about you. For example, you can take out a half-page ad in a local health magazine, where your ad has been designed to showcase what you offer and tout your skills. You paid for that ad and essentially, you are saying things about yourself. When a PR firm works on your behalf, they send media things that may get turned into articles and feature stories on the news.

When that happens, they are giving you the promotion and they are saying things about your office.

Public relations firms do something that you can also do, which is to send out regular press releases, media alerts, and help to keep a good relationship with the media. Why keep those good relationships? Well, when a health reporter goes to do an article where they may need to interview an orthodontist, you want to be the one they turn to. That's free publicity that you will benefit from. You don't have to have a PR firm handle these tasks either; sending out press releases and building relationships with your local health reporters is something your office can do. Just be sure to know the guidelines when it comes to writing and submitting professional press releases.

One quick word on the idea of press releases, because many people are confused by them. You don't have to wait to send out a press release only when you are hiring a new doctor or purchasing a new building. While those are legitimate reasons to send out press releases, there are many, many other opportunities that you should consider. Often times, health reporters get their story ideas from the press releases that come their way. As an orthodontist, throughout the year you can send out releases that focus on such things as "5 Things to Know About Do It Yourself Braces" or "What Every Parent Needs to Know About Oral Piercings." Every Halloween and Easter, you can send out a list of doctor-approved treats for those with braces. There are many ideas, angles and opportunities to get your name out there and help solidify yourself as an expert in your market.

In chapter 12, we will look more deeply at owning your media platform, which is a tremendously beneficial area and deserves your attention. If you want more media exposure and assistance with public relations and publishing your book, contact my friends at Advantage Media | Forbes books. They have helped countless clients of mine to establish their practices as the trusted authority in their market. Learn more at www.AdvantageFamily.com

On the other end of the spectrum in public relations is the area of taking care of the top 100-150 people that you want to keep in your orbit. These are the people you want to always maintain contact with at least twice per year.

There are a variety of ways that you can take care of this list, but one that you should consider is CRM software, which stands for Customer Relationship Management.

CRM programs are designed to help you keep track of these 100-150 people. You can add notes, reminders, important dates and build an automated sequence for staying in touch with these important individuals within your orbit. It will track your history with the person. For example, if you know the dentist across town who sends you referrals has a collection of classic cars, you can add that bit of trivia to the database. That way, when you pull up his name, you are quickly reminded what the person likes. You can even add in their birthday, business anniversary date, or any other pertinent information that you feel may be helpful later on.

Every time you have contact with that person, especially since your goal is at least a couple of times per year, the information will be recorded in the system. Every couple of months, you can run a quick report to see who hasn't been given any attention lately. Then you know who to set your sights on. CRM programs are an easy way to help keep things organized, helping you to have the information you need at your fingertips. It doesn't have to be anything elaborate, and they are well worth the investment.

When you keep in contact with people on a regular basis, you will help to build a stronger relationship. These relationships are what will grow your practice. From the reporters, you will gain media stories, image branding, and help to be established as an expert in the area. From the non-media relationships, such as those you will maintain with dentists and other professionals in your area, you will ultimately gain referrals. You will gain a steady stream of influence, which is the real currency of every successful orthodontic practice.

Another thing you will gain from each of these areas is trust, which is the foundation of every relationship. When people trust you, they will speak well of you and want to refer others to your office. They can only learn to trust you if you take the time to cultivate the relationship. Again, don't assume that it's their job to pick up the phone and make a connection. You want and need these connections, so let the ego take a back seat and just focus on doing what you need to in order to keep them going, and to strengthen them.

Picking One

Public relations is one of the 15 areas that you can choose to own to help propel your practice to ultimate success. I can tell you right now that I can go to any town in America and to most countries around the world, and I could pick one of these 15 core competencies and find someone who is doing it better than everyone else in that market. They have simply chosen to own that particular area and they stand out for it.

When you own a particular core competency, you will be far and above others in your market. You will stand out as the clear winner and category leader in that particular market. You don't have to own them all, but you do have to find one and do it so well that the people will flock to you. You are like a magnet. Right now, I could walk into your town, go around the main square, and find someone who owns a business who's the best at networking. And I can assure you that he's killing it. Maybe he owns a car dealership, or a real estate office. Then I could go and find someone who is the best at hiring good people. He's got the best paralegals around, the best associates, and that person is killing it. Then I can go and find the person in retail who is the best at sales. You get the idea here.

Maybe your thing is that everyone loves being around you. Maybe you are the networking guy, or you are great at putting the best people together. Perhaps people come to you and say "Do you know anyone who could help me with this real estate deal?" And you are the one who connects these two and now, you are the glue that binds relationships. Maybe that's you. Doesn't matter what it is that you choose and are great at, but you have to choose one area and you have to be the one who is killing it.

Public relations is great area to own if you are someone who enjoys networking, is more introverted, and understands the importance of maintaining relationships. You have to want to keep at least those 100 people in your orbit, do the work that it takes to pull it off, and do it well. You have to do it so well that people see you as someone who is great at maintaining contact, remembering and thinking of people, and who can take the responsibility for keeping people in contact, rather than waiting for others to do it.

You care about your reputation and how people in the public view your office. One of the great things about the area of public relations is that it focuses on protecting and enhancing that reputation with the community. You are more in control of the connections being made and can help keep them in your favor. Public relations will focus on making your practice and you look good, which will build trust and strengthen relationships. When that happens, you will end up with more referrals, respect, and a clear path toward huge success.

Owning It

When you choose to own the area of public relations, you will have great synergy with all those around you. The focus of your office will be to cultivate great relationships with local dentists, hygienists, pediatricians, health reporters, vendors, and more. That's a positive thing to do, and when you live your life in a positive way, good things are bound to happen. Choosing an area that will put you front and center in working on creating great relationships is not only one that will be beneficial, but it can also be fun. You will have a variety of people who you network with, and will know people from multiple fields. It's networking at its finest. Owning the area of public relations takes networking one step further, so you are no longer just exchanging business cards. Instead, you are taking steps every year to make sure that those important people remain in your orbit. That's a situation that will help you create friends, build trustworthy relationships, and will lead to respect and referrals.

Without even realizing it, you already have a relationship with the public. Chances are, you don't give it much thought, and therefore don't go out of your way to ensure that your connections are great and the important people stay in your orbit. By owning public relations, you will take measures that will lead to people having a more favorable opinion of you and your office. It's already there, you might as well weed and water it.

"Publicity is absolutely critical. A good PR story is infinitely more effective than a front page ad." - Richard Branson

---

CHAPTER TWELVE
MEDIA PLATFORM

"Don't be afraid to give up the good to go for the great." -John D. Rockefeller

When you pick up a magazine or daily newspaper, do you ever wonder where the story ideas come from? I'm not referring to things like breaking news and headlines about what's going on in the world. I'm talking about the stories that people find of interest, that are helpful in their lives, covering such topics as health issues, how to weed and feed your lawn, or what's the best way to shop for new flooring. If you haven't thought about it, you are not alone.

Most people look through magazines, newspapers, and online media outlets, never giving it any thought at all. They may watch hours of television news or listen to talk radio shows and not once wonder about what prompted a particular story of interest. Believe it or not, a lot of those stories are started by people just like you and me, who want to get particular information into the media so that it reaches the masses.

That's right, what you don't know about media relations is most likely holding your practice back in a big way. When you learn more about how it works, you will be able to leverage that power to help grow your practice. If you decide to own the area of media relations, then the sky is the limit. You will have media at your fingertips, so you can reach a large audience on a regular basis. This route to reaching people comes with numerous benefits, which is why we have mastered it in our office and use it regularly.

When you learn about media relations, including the benefits and how to go about making it a part of your practice, you will wonder why you never did it before. You don't have to be a large company like Disney or Apple to use media relations to your benefit. And trust me, they use it a lot and benefit from it greatly. You can use the same tactics on a smaller scale, and gain some fantastic results that will help your practice thrive.

How News is Created

When it comes to stories of interest, such as those in the health and lifestyle section of your newspaper, in parenting magazines, and on the health segments on your television news, many of them are generated by everyday people. It may seem as though the writers and reporters are scouring for things to write about, and sometimes they are, but that's one of the perks of focusing on media relations.

When you focus on media relations, you are giving the writers and reporters ideas to focus on. Rather than reporters and producers always coming up with article and segment ideas, you feed them great content and make their jobs easier. You help them out by giving them ideas, as well as some of the information they can use in the news segments. This is done through a variety of ways, including using press releases and media alerts.

A newspaper might receive hundreds of press releases each day, but they are always looking for things to cover, so they will pick some of them to use. If you own media relations, you will maintain a great relationship with the writers, editors, and reporters, and that will help boost the chances that your information is used more often. Stories in the media are often generated through this age-old process, and once you learn how to own it, it will work great for you as well. You would be surprised at how many media outlets are actively trying to find content each week, giving you an edge when you systematically send them interesting content.

If a reporter uses a story idea, press release, media alert, or content that was sent into them, then that person has helped to create news or content that will be used by that media outlet. They may use the whole thing or just a part of it, but you should get a mention out of it at least. Often times you will get much

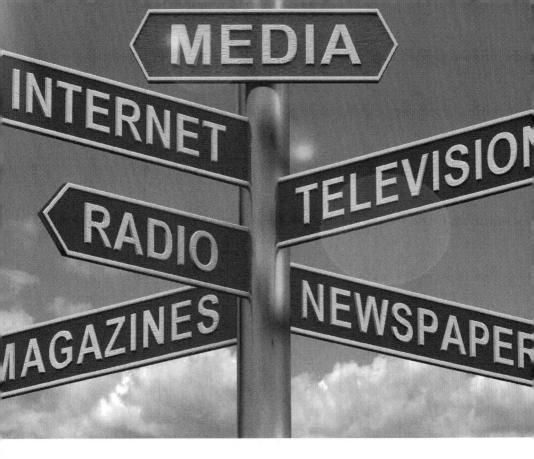

more than that, and will be surprised at the amount of what we refer to as free exposure you can get when you focus on media relations.

Getting that exposure is thought of as free media, because it's something that you earned by your media relations management. It's not something that you paid for, such as advertising. With media exposure, you don't usually pay for the exposure, you have just earned it through your efforts of providing useful and timely information and often times by maintaining a good relationship with the reporter or media outlet.

There's no limit to the places where you can send stories and segment ideas. You have open access to local newspapers, magazines, television, online sites, and more. Every one of those outlets has a tremendous need for subject matter to fill all of their air time and keep feeding the content monster. Day after day, month after month, that can become a monumental task for them, so they appreciate and need people to send them things for consideration. Quite honestly, it's a win-win situation for everyone, because they need the content and you need the exposure.

Getting it Done

Many people who keep up with what I do know that I do a lot of content marketing. I do this in a variety of ways, covering all bases. I have books, reports, recipes, and I even get my share of time on the television. All of this is systematic, which is something that most people don't realize. How we've gotten on TV, how we've gotten on the covers of magazines, and how we've produced our own repots, is all systematic. We now produce our magazines and newsletters, with all of it being very intentional.

Nothing we've done has been by mistake. It's all thought out, planned, and we take action to help make it happen. Our goal is to educate people. Think about all of the new apps popping up with local hospitals and medical centers. Mobile telemedicine doctors are now calling on your Smartphone. Things like this are all intentional and all up and coming ways of delivering content to a targeted group of people. Maybe you will be the next person to think of some version or app that will help people in your area with the health and orthodontic information they need, right at their fingertips. Your app can be complete with reminders, helpful articles, brace friendly recipes, local store and restaurant discounts, and more. Like Walt Disney liked to say, if you can dream it, you can do it.

Maybe you will be the person to think of some app version that allows us to show up at your house and do your Invisalign ClinCheck with a GoPro camera, so that you can look at the patient remotely. Content delivery and patient interaction like that may seem crazy when you first hear it, but when you give it some thought it's easy to see that this could absolutely be the future. Imagine how great remote check-ups could be for you and your patients. There's nothing more convenient for them, which helps to push past the excuses. It may seem crazy, but my bet is on the fact that it's coming our way. We've already explored it.

I get a good amount of media attention, and I assure you that it's not because I'm the bee's knees. I'm an orthodontist and no different than all of you. Truth be told, I'm not even that charismatic. I'm actually kind of shy most of the time. So it's not that I have some amazing personality that makes me stand out and get media attention. The reason I get a lot of attention from the media is because we've attached ourselves to a higher sense of purpose. Maybe that's your thing for the coming year, too.

It's all about attaching yourself to something beyond yourself. Maybe you are will own the area of media platform and you will be the best at getting media attention. Or maybe you are the best at events or innovation in the field. I don't care which one it is, but you have to pick one of the areas that you are going to own and be the best at doing it. Own media relations and you will stand out as a rock star in your market.

If you own the area of philanthropy, you will get a lot of attention for that. I've had many orthodontists help me treat countless kids through Smiles Change Lives. I love that the program changes the lives of a lot of kids, but at the same time we help to grow our practices. I care about your practice and want you to be wildly successful, which is why I try to share everything I've learned about how to run a highly successful orthodontic practice. Owning this area can make a world of difference for your practice and generate a considerable amount of free publicity as well.

Why it's Great

As you can see, I'm a big fan of having a strong media platform. There are many benefits that come from having media connections, and far more if it's an area that you have decided to own. In the prior chapter, I explained the difference between advertising and public relations. If you recall, advertising is something you are going to pay for, such as an ad placement in a magazine. On the other side, public relations (which is your media platform) is content and media mentions that you have earned, rather than having paid for them. You are not paying a reporter to work on a story angle that you suggest. You don't pay a newspaper to print an article you wrote about the best way to care for braces. And you also don't pay to be interviewed on the TV news when they do a story on pediatric oral health.

Getting these things to happen takes place because of your efforts. You write the materials and you get them out to those you feel should have them. If you maintain good relationships with those in the media and you continuously offer them good quality content and ideas, you will be rewarded with being featured in their segments, articles, and news stories.

When you have an item that appears in the news, and it's good content and information that helps people, you will help to do a number of things for you and your practice. You will build your credibility and become seen as an expert in the area. You will become the go-to person when someone has a question about orthodontics. It's great when you become the person they think of when they need a quote or interview. That's free publicity, and you want this all day, every day, because it pays off in big ways. All the free publicity also helps with your image branding and networking. You will be surprised at how it helps people begin to recognize you, your office name, and in the varied people you will meet to network with as a result of the media attention.

Who among us can't use more public credibility, image branding, and being seen as an expert in the area? We can all benefit from that. Owning the media platform area will help you to grow your practice. Not only will potential patients see you and want to call your office, but they will refer you to others because they have seen you and know you have the credibility to be interviewed by the media. You will also get new referrals from dentists. They will see you in the media and the referrals will follow. Being in the media this way helps you to manage your reputation and that of your practice, so you will ensure that you have a favorable reputation in the community.

There's another area that many people overlook when it comes to having a great media platform. When you gain the attention of being an expert and respected office in the community, there's a good chance you are also going to recruit the best talent in the field. When you need to hire people, you will have the best people clamoring to get a position at your office. When you get the best talent in your area, you know your team is going to excel and so is your office.

Many people have a desperate fear of public speaking, but being in the media can also get you invited to do speaking engagements. If you fear speaking on camera to reporters, you fear giving a presentation to local dentists, or you would rather crawl under a rock than to give a speech at a conference, there is something you can do about it. This is a fear that you can overcome and even excel at. Don't miss out on the great opportunities that owning the area of media platform offers because you fear public speaking. Rather, seek to change those fears by learning how to overcome them. Join a local Toastmasters group to learn how to feel comfortable with public speaking. The benefits far outweigh your fears, and it's something you can overcome with practice.

The Many Ways

One of the great things about owning the area of media relations is that you have a wide variety of avenues to explore. Here are some ideas that I utilize and some ideas on how to go about implementing them:

Press releases and media alerts. One of the oldest and most popular tools people use are press releases and media alerts. While they sound like they may be two of the same, they are in fact not the same thing. A press release is written in the style of an article. In fact, it is an article and should be written in a manner that if the media outlet wanted to pick it up from the page you sent them, they should be able to paste it right into their print magazine, newspaper or online. It's something that is ready to be used in its current form. It also serves the purpose of giving a heads up about something that is happening or has happened. Details can be pulled from it to use in stories. The reporter can choose to use the whole thing as it is, gather info from it, or take bits and pieces from it to use in their segment. They decide how they want to use it.

Media alerts are more of a factual piece that is going to provide reporters with the who, what, where, when, and why. It's not written in an article format, it tends to be more of a list of details about something that is taking place that you want the media to know about. These are sent out to a variety of media outlets, including television, newspapers, magazines, local websites and more.

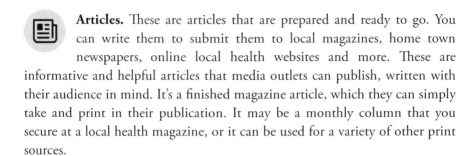

Articles. These are articles that are prepared and ready to go. You can write them to submit them to local magazines, home town newspapers, online local health websites and more. These are informative and helpful articles that media outlets can publish, written with their audience in mind. It's a finished magazine article, which they can simply take and print in their publication. It may be a monthly column that you secure at a local health magazine, or it can be used for a variety of other print sources.

Educational articles. These are articles that you have printed up to look like magazine quality articles, but they are distributed by your office. We have many of these great articles that cover a variety of topics. They look, feel, and read like a magazine article, where we are the expert source. We give these to our patients at various stages in treatment, so that they have their questions answered in an interesting way and they have the option of passing them on to others. We also put these articles in our new patient kit that goes out to every patient that makes an appointment.

Pitches. You are an expert in your field. You are an orthodontist with years of experience, your own practice, and you would make a great expert to be interviewed for segments that relate to your field. Only the reporters in your area have no clue, because you are not on their radar or in their orbit. This is where media pitches come into play. A media pitch, simply put, is a one-page write-up that introduces reporters in your area to who you are, what you know, what you can speak about and that you'd love to be considered as an expert source the next time they need an orthodontist to interview. Send that out to all of the reporters in your area and you will get some attention from it. I've known people who were contacted back for television interviews, to be quoted in print news and more.

It's important to interject here a word of caution about what you send out to the media. The media pitch is a tool that sells you to the reporter as an expert in the field that they can call upon. The media alert is a fact-driven document, such as giving the details about an event you are hosting. But the content you send out, such as the articles and press releases, cannot be sales pitches. If they are sales pitches and merely come across as a sales pitch for your office, they will quickly be discarded. Then your credibility will be toast and they will learn to not look at anything else you send their way. That's the opposite of what you want to happen.

When you send out press releases, articles, and other content that can be used, it needs to be written in a professional manner that is informative and not a sales pitch for your office. Yes, you are the source that is being quoted, so there's a plug for you, but beyond that the article needs to focus on being interesting and informative to the reader. It's not about selling you and your office to the reader, it's about giving them helpful info and them seeing your name mingled in. Press releases have a boilerplate at the bottom, where you will mention your office, and there may be some times when a call to action makes sense. But overall, don't go in with guns blazing and a hard sales pitch, because that will have a negative outcome.

Owning It
If you choose to own the area of media platforms, you will need to choose the best person to manage it. Some people hire a public relations expert to handle these tasks, while others handle it in-house, putting one person in charge. You can also do a combination of the two. You have to see what works for your office and what you are the most comfortable with, but whoever is going to take this on needs to know how each of the media tools work and how to manage them effectively and efficiently.

Owning the area of media platform is a great way to get your name out there, build your office recognition and get interviewed on topics in your field. There are many benefits that come from it. This is one more area for you to consider that will help bring in more referrals and grow your office. In today's technology-driven world, there are more media opportunities than ever before. They are everywhere. Owning this area means tapping into them to boost your office in numerous ways.

There are many ideas that you can send out to the media. Take on the task of coming up with writing down 10 ideas per day. If you do this for one month, it will change your life.

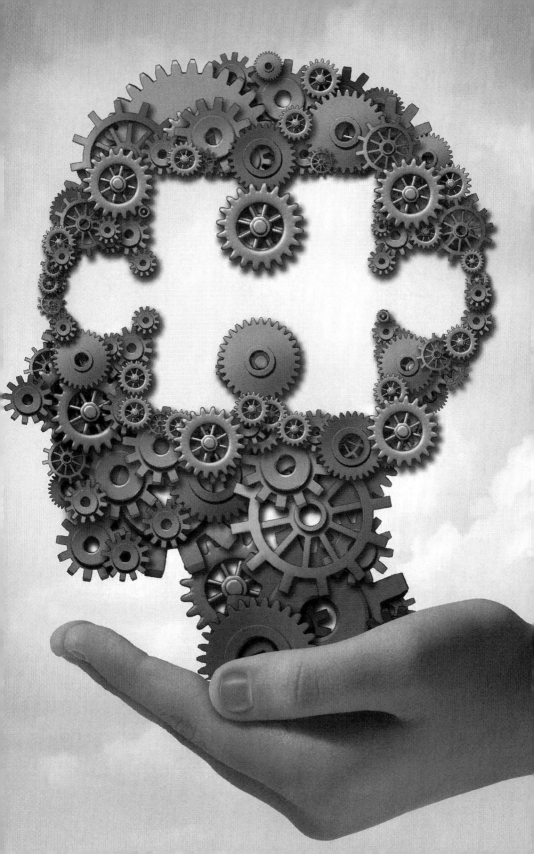

CHAPTER THIRTEEN
EDUCATION

"Get a good idea and stay with it. Dog it, and work at it until it's done right." – Walt Disney

Each of the 15 core competency areas in this book have made it in here because I've seen firsthand that 95% of orthodontist offices are missing them. I've learned a lot from running my own practice, but I've also learned a massive amount of good information by working with other orthodontists in consulting and by having thousands of hours of secret shopper videos. In other words, you could say that I've owned the area of knowing what it takes to run a highly successful orthodontist practice.

I made that my goal and did the research that it took to get here. I have seen that offices consistently drop the ball in these 15 areas. Choosing to own just one of them and then doing it better than it's ever been done before is going to put you far ahead of the competition. The beauty in this, however, is that even in the areas that you don't end up owning, you will find that improvements are made just by reading this book.

Once you have become aware of each issue in this book, there's no turning back. You can't unlearn the information, and even if you never own it, you will likely make some improvements in each area. Once you combine making some improvements in numerous areas and owning one and doing it better than anyone else, you will see some amazing things happen in your practice.

Education Abounds

Have you ever stopped to think about the wealth of information that you and your office can offer the world? As a professional in the field, you have a vast amount of education and experience, as does your team. When it comes down to it, your practice has a ton of information that can be used to educate a wide variety of people.

Owning the area of education means taking all that information and getting it out to those who need it, and doing so in a professional and interesting manner. It means putting it out there in a better way than anyone else is doing it in your area. When you do that, you appear to be the absolute expert when it comes to people being educated on all things orthodontics. There are a lot of benefits to be the one who is going to educate the public about orthodontists.

For starters, when you are the definitive expert on orthodontics in your area, people will turn to you for advice, with questions, to provide you with referrals, to be their expert source and so much more. You will become the person people turn to anytime they think about orthodontics. This is a good thing, because it will bring with it great networking opportunities, educational outreach opportunities, and you guessed it, more referrals. When you are seen as the expert in the area, you are going to get a lot of referrals come your way as a result.

At our practice, we have used the area of education for years to help us reach out to a variety of people, and the results have been great. Never underestimate the power of great content and what it can do for you when it's in the hands of the right people.

You have probably heard the saying "content is king" before, and for good reason. People want and crave content, but not any content. It has to be good content that is useful to them. Consumers can spot shoddy content a mile away and they will avoid it. In fact, if it's not good, then it may even have a damaging effect on your reputation. If you own the area of education, the content you produce needs to be top-notch, professional and it needs to offer your audience information they can use. When you do that, they will come back for more and remember your name.

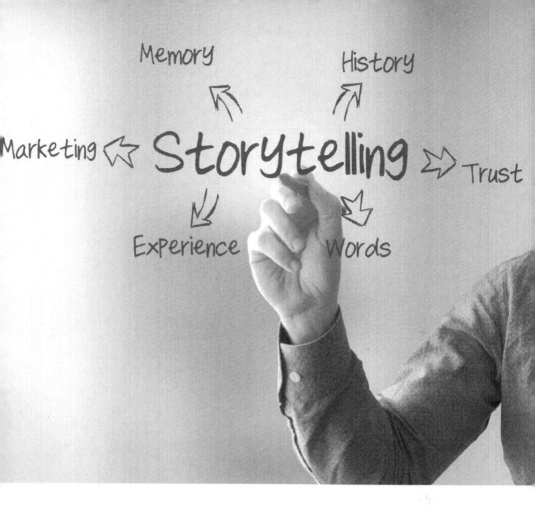

When you offer your area great educational materials, content, workshops and more, you will increase your reach, generate referrals, gain authority in the field, encourage engagement, add value to your practice and build your brand awareness. People have questions and they need answers. If you are the one to answer those questions, and do so in a way that resonates with them, your office will reap the rewards.

By producing content and campaigns to help educate others, you are able to capture your voice in them. This helps people to learn more about your brand. Everything you send out, create and offer in the form of education has essentially been stamped with your own identification. People feel like they get to know you better because your voice comes through in each educational item that you put out. After all, your voice is your personality. What happens when people get to know you and your personality more? Well, as I like to remind people, referrals are largely based upon relationships. When you take the time to build relationships, you will without a doubt get more referrals. Your voice resonating throughout all of the educational work you do helps people get to know your personality, which helps establish, strengthen and maintain a relationship.

Something else you can add to what you put out there and do for education is authenticity. If you haven't focused on building your brand image yet, this is the time to do it. Your brand image and authenticity will be present in everything you do. You want to make sure that it all sends the right message about you, your personality and your brand image.

Owning the area of education means taking what you know and helping people understand it. You know a lot and have a wealth of education to share with others. You might be surprised at just how many different ways you can use education, producing content and a wide variety of campaigns, to offer bits and pieces to your community, to other dentists, to hygienists and more.

Who Cares

At first thought, you might think patients are the only target market for consuming educational content. While they are certainly one of the areas you can focus on and should, there are other areas as well. There are many ways that you can distribute educational content in order to help your practice.

Let's take a look at each of the ways and how you can tap into them to achieve the best results.

Patients. *Of course, your patients are one of the main areas to include when owning the area of education.* Your prospective patients, current patients and past ones are all potential areas to consider and tap into. People have questions, they are curious, and sometimes they don't even know they want or need something until the information is presented to them. Providing them with the educational information they need can be huge for your practice. You can do this in a variety of ways, such as producing articles, brochures and welcome packets that offer the information they need when starting and continuing treatment. You can give them information every step of the way as they go through various stages of treatment. There are so many options here, including giving them braces-friendly recipes, newsletters, frequently asked questions and more. You can offer the educational information on our website, social media channels and in person.

We also live in a time when people love to watch videos, giving you another option for providing patients with educational information. Creating short, yet insightful, videos to post on your website and social media channels is a good way to help further your reach.

Parents. *Putting educational information out there for parents is crucial.* They have questions, concerns and often times need to know the benefits of getting their children treatment. Most parents have no idea at what age a child should first see an orthodontist or the different types of treatment and financing options available to them. These are the things they need answers to if you have hopes of getting them to bring their children into your office for an evaluation or to begin treatment.

Parents can also benefit from some of the information that is provided to patients. They will find it helpful to get tips on foods that can be eaten with braces and those that can be avoided, what to do if a bracket breaks on a Sunday afternoon or things they can do to help their child if they are having some discomfort. Parents often need the information that offers the facts, and especially the benefits about why having a great smile is so important and how it can have a major impact on their child's life as they grow up. From letting them know the best time to begin orthodontics to the benefits of having an evaluation at an early age, there are plenty of educational opportunities for parents. Some parents may need child thumb sucking advice, while others may not realize that protruding teeth are more prone to being chipped. Information for parents can also be delivered in a wide variety of ways, including magazine articles, books, brochures, social media posts and videos, to name a few.

You can also hold informative educational seminars and workshops for parents, where some of the most common issues in orthodontics can be addressed, giving you a chance to provide them with information and meet them face-to-face at the same time. Educational information for parents can be in your office, online, given to the school nurse, on a stand in the pediatrician offices and dispersed in a wide variety of ways. Get creative in considering the many places where you can get more information into the hands of parents, by having it available where they frequent.

Referring doctors. *These centers of influence are gold to your office and you want to do everything you can to keep them in your orbit.* You also want to do what you can to keep them supplied with the information they need to give their patients regarding orthodontics. But it doesn't stop there, because you want to provide them with information that can be useful to them and their staff. Holding educational workshops and seminars is a good way to keep them up to date, give them information about what's new and give them the tools and answers they need for their patients. Hosting such events gives you an opportunity to keep each of them at arm's length and to provide them with useful information. At least a couple of times per year, aim to have a workshop for referring doctors, where you provide a catered dinner and present some useful information. Be sure to make a point of speaking with each of them individually to further your networking and relationship building.

You can also hold periodic educational workshops for the hygienists, nurses and additional dental office staff, so that they are better able to answer questions that they receive. You would be surprised at how many will be happy to attend a catered workshop, where they can earn some CEU's, have a chance to win some prizes, and learn something they can use. Each one is an opportunity to shake a hand, make a contact and start the relationship building. Webinars are another great way to hold educational outreach events to get the information in the hands of doctors, hygienists and other professionals who may be able to gain from the knowledge and also be in a position to send your office referrals.

Community. *The people in your community can benefit greatly from having their orthodontic questions answered.* This can be done through writing articles that get printed in local magazines, newspapers and online. It can also be done by giving talks on orthodontic topics and providing the community with information they can use. Consider holding an event once or twice per year that is just for the community to come and learn all about orthodontics, explaining to them what can be done and the benefits of treatment. Your talk could be given at the local elementary school, with parents being invited, or it could be held at a community health fair, where you are a guest speaker. There are plenty of ways to give out educational information to the community at large, whether you are setting up a booth at a health fair, guest speaking, or holding your own events and inviting people to come learn more. You can own the area of education and still use the section on live events in order to get some tips on the various ways that you can reach the public and meet face-to-face. Just be sure to keep education in mind, so that whatever you are doing you will be providing them with something they can use and that will help them in their lives.

Media. There is a lot that you can take from the section on owning the media to use here when reaching out to reporters. You might not solely focus on owning the area of media, but when you own education it makes perfect sense to have it be part of that package.

The media is always looking for information to provide their readers and viewers. They need articles, story ideas, and experts to interview for news segments. *When you own the area of education, you will become the best person around at providing them with the materials and answers they need.* You can supply them with educational story ideas, articles that are ready to be used just as they are sent in and you can become their go-to expert when they need an orthodontic expert to quote. You can send them materials and you can also hold educational outreach events for reporters. Imagine what you would get from hosting a catered breakfast for health reporters and providing them with some educational orthodontic tips that they can use.

Even if you have never given much thought to hosting events, you'll be the only one in your town who attempts and you'll likely be pleased with the results. Establishing and maintaining a good relationship with the media has serious benefits for your practice. It's always a good idea to network with those in the media and to become their go-to person for all things related to orthodontics.

Thinking beyond. Orthodontic educational materials have additional places where they can be used and distributed. Thinking beyond just the outlets listed will give you an opportunity to expand your reach and tap into new markets.

When you own the area of education, your mode of thinking will always be focused on what you can provide others to help educate and inform them. You will think of new topics, new avenues and materials and how to expand your pool of who receives these materials. Again, you will become the best there is in your area at providing orthodontic educational materials and information.

Targeting Your Market

When it comes to providing educational and informational content and activities, it is important to always keep your market in mind. The materials you use, whether you are creating content that will be distributed or you are organizing a workshop, should always be geared toward the audience. You wouldn't have the same focus for moms attending a workshop to learn about braces for their children as you would having an educational event for local dentists. Owning the area of education, you will become a master planner when it comes to identifying target markets, and ensuring that materials have been created for each specific market. This means you will have a lot of different topics, but they are geared toward different segments of the population.

Without targeting your market and using materials to match, your message will be lost and you will not reap the benefits that owning this core competency can bring. When you take the time to target your market and match the materials expertly, you will maximize your return on investment, and it will be well worth your efforts. Once you have targeted your market, getting creative with your approach will only help your results.

When targeting consumer markets, it's also important to avoid using jargon and terms that patients and parents don't understand. While dentists are comfortable reading industry terms, there are many parents who are not. Ideally, materials for parents and the general public should be written using terms and at a level they can easily understand. If you are unsure if it's written at a level that parents would feel comfortable with and can relate to, have one or two parents do a test read for you and get their honest feedback. The nature and style of the materials should be treated with a high level of importance. Every piece of content has your stamp of approval and image, so make sure it's exactly what you want to put into the marketplace.

Owning the area of education, it is also beneficial for you to keep up with trends and changes in the field. You can keep tabs on new products, the trends that are going on with teens and braces and any new research about orthodontics that comes out that you could share with parents and dentists. Create a Google Alert for these areas. Make it a point to buy relevant magazines and books consumed by these market segments. This further helps you serve a larger population and will solidify you as an expert in the field. Your image will be that of someone who knows the industry inside and out and has all the info that everyone else needs to know.

Owning It

Imagine being that one orthodontist in your entire area that nails it when it comes to providing the whole community with educational materials, educational outreach events and more. What would something like that mean to your practice? It would mean a lot, because you would be owning it to the point where you do it better than it's ever been done before. You would stand out as an expert in the field and be the first person people think of when they want orthodontic information.

When you can consistently provide people with relevant and valuable information, you build trust. Every relationship is built on a foundation of trust. Once you have trust, you can grow that relationship and that's when you will see referrals continue to grow. With more referrals, your practice will thrive and become highly successful, regardless of market swings.

Being the person that others turn to when they want reliable, honest, and helpful information will always be a good thing. No, make that a great thing. Information and knowledge is power. It's a power that can lead your practice down the road to more referrals, more brand recognition and a lot more success.

"If you are not taking care of your customer, your competitor will." - Bob Hooey

---

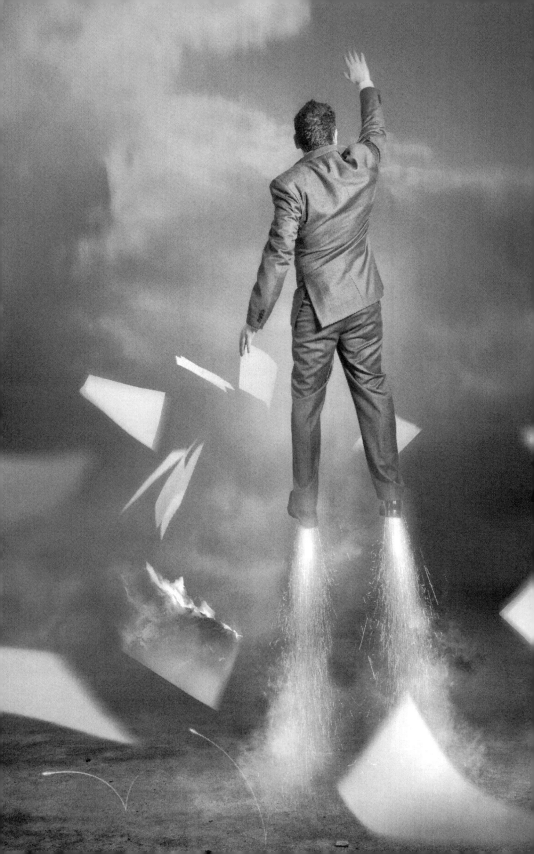

CHAPTER FOURTEEN
TRANSPORTATION

"Innovation distinguishes between a leader and a follower." – Steve Jobs

When you think about the word transportation, you conjure up images of vehicles, airplanes, and other such things. While those are transportation, they are not exactly the type of transportation that I'm referring to here. Those forms of transportation, however, are representative of the idea behind what this chapter is about. Transportation keeps things moving along, expedited, swiftly moving from one place to another. In essence, that's what owning transportation would mean for your orthodontic practice, too.

There are various ways that we use the concept of transportation in our office. I've seen how these things can help keep the office moving along swiftly, helping to avoid many of the roadblocks and snags that get other offices hung up. We've gotten to this point, of course, by learning along the way that there are better and more efficient ways of doing things. I've also learned a great deal about the importance of transportation by watching the many secret shopper videos that we've collected. These videos demonstrate the most common areas where practices get held up, creating a traffic jam of sorts.

When you have these backups and traffic jams, they hold your practice back from seeing more people, meeting more people's needs, and from being as efficient as you possibly can be. Efficiency and swiftness is going to keep your office moving in the right direction. It's necessary so that you don't become stagnant and stuck in a rut. Working in consulting over the years, I have also seen the issues through the lens of other orthodontists. I hear what their hang-ups are, whether or not they have been able to identify them, and what they do about them once they see there's a problem and realize there is a better way.

Often times, we tend to get hung up doing things the way we do, simply because we don't yet know a better, more efficient way. We continue to do something the way we do, because that's the way it's always been done. Only when we question this are we able to identify areas that can be improved. The improvements we make in our office and in how we work with our patients will always pay off. Nobody is perfect, and we should always strive to make improvements that will benefit our patients. Anything that benefits our patients will benefit our entire practice. Making such improvements is a win-win situation that is well worth the investment.

There are numerous ways you can own the area of transportation in order to help your patients, and in turn help your entire practice. When you nail the area of transportation, or any one particular area, you will be surprised at just how much it does to help propel more growth in your practice. As I've explained, you don't have to own every area. You may find that exhausting, and it is definitely more difficult to master several areas. But you do have to pick one of these areas and own it. Doing so will be huge for your practice and you will wonder why you never did it before. Yes, it's that powerful.

Three of the main areas of transportation that we focus on in our practice are having multiple locations, our clear retainer delivery system and having a great referral network. If you own the area of transportation, you may want to focus on these areas, or others, but this gives you an idea of what you can do with the area and how important it can be to your practice.

Multiple Locations

Most orthodontists have one or two locations. And they don't usually question that at all. They open an office, serve the people who decide to make the drive and then keep doing the same thing year after year. But do you realize how many people you are missing out on treating simply because your office is too far away? Let's be honest about the fact that most people don't want to drive very far to go to an orthodontist, even if they have heard good things about

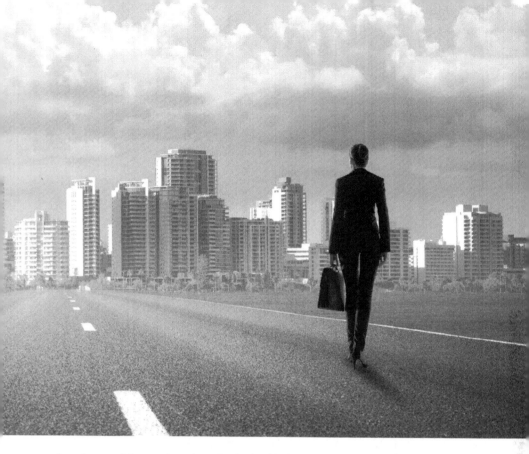

that doctor. It's not that they don't think it's worth it or that they don't like to drive. The problem is that we just live in a day and age when people are busier than ever before.

Every parent who needs to get their child to orthodontic appointments already has a long list of things they have to do. Their child plays multiple sports, has after-school activities, homework and a host of other responsibilities. Many families don't even have time to eat dinner together regularly. When they do get a little extra time, they don't want to spend it going to an orthodontist on the other side of town. They will find one closer to home, because they cherish their time. They know they need that extra time for something else and they don't want the stress of trying to make the drive over to you.

When this happens, and trust me it happens a lot, you are missing out on a lot of patients who you would otherwise be seeing. It may even be the one major thing holding your practice back from reaching the level of success that you dream of having. It's simply about the logistics. Your geographical location, as much as you like or hate it, is going to have an impact on the amount of patients you can see and treat. Your office is just simply out of reach for many people who would like to see you, but only have so much time in their life and have a ton of things they need to try to do with it.

This is why it's so important to consider having multiple locations. When we took the leap to having multiple locations, our success rate went through the roof. Today, we have four offices spread throughout the area, so that we are able to provide treatment to everyone in our market. Geographic location is one thing that will not hold us back from reaching everyone in our area. We have made it very easy for them to reach us, no matter where they live in town.

This was all well planned out. We strategically identified where each office would be located, so that it's easy for people to reach us. In fact, rather than expecting our patients to come to us, we essentially went to them. Knowing that people don't want to make a long drive to see the orthodontist, we brought the orthodontist closer to them. People love that we have four offices, making it very efficient for them to choose us for their treatment.

In strategically choosing where to place your office locations, you will open your practice up to a larger market. Accommodate people the best you can. But you can go another step to help make it even more convenient. For example, at our offices, we are open from 7 a.m. to 7 p.m. on school days. We do this because we absolutely know that some people don't want to miss school or work to come in for an appointment. This gives them the ability to make appointments with zero inconvenience and makes it easy for them to say yes to our office. People greatly appreciate it, and without a doubt we get a lot of patients who otherwise might go to a competitor. Parents can only take so much time off of work and kids can only miss so much school. When they see you have an office close to them and you have made it so that school and work won't need to be missed, you have created a winning combination that many parents can't resist.

We also take it even further in our multiple locations, making it even more convenient for patients. We offer Saturday appointments. Most doctors don't want to offer weekend appointments, but many parents crave them so that they don't interfere with the other long list of things going on in their lives. We offer appointments every Saturday, and have many patients who take advantage of it. Our flexibility in having multiple locations and in the days and hours that we offer appointments is very attractive to parents who have kids that need treatment.

There are additional things we do at our office locations that further entice people to choose us for their treatment. These include offering a guarantee for "drop-in" appointments, and that we offer free second opinions. Both of these things bring comfort to patients, and by having multiple locations we are convenient enough that it makes these perks a reality for them. Guaranteed drop-in appointments wouldn't be nearly as attractive if we had one location on the far side of town. People know that by us having convenient locations they will truly be able to use that service if and when they need to use it.

There are great benefits of having multiple locations. Not only is it more convenient, but it's great for your office's professionalism and public image. Just about everyone would agree that multiple locations is a clear sign of success. The public sees that, realizes you have a successful practice, and that happens because you must be good. Having four locations, it's hard for people to not have heard of us. Having multiple locations is great for your professionalism and public image, showing people that you have a major presence in the area.

Finally, having multiple locations is going to do great things for your revenue numbers. Consider what you are doing at your office and then imagine what that would look like times three or four. It is possible with some strategic planning, and when you own the area of transportation that is exactly what you will be doing. You will do it better than it's ever been done before in your area, and you will earn a reputation and public image as the orthodontist above all others. With multiple locations, you expand your reach. We even offer pediatric dentistry at our offices, which adds more convenience, and makes for a smooth transition for those who need to get orthodontic treatment. They don't need to go elsewhere, they will keep coming to the same office that they are familiar with in order to get orthodontic treatment for their children.

Clear Retainer Delivery

Being able to expedite clear retainer delivery is a must for the orthodontic office that wants to keep things flowing. Without a doubt, clear retainers are going to continue to need to be ordered and replaced. Whether they are wearing out, discoloring, or being lost, they are commonly needed. Since it is something that is so commonly needed, it is a process that should be well automated.

Being able to take your clear retainer delivery process and keep it smooth, automated and swift will be a great service to both your patients and your office. No longer will your office be hung up on the ordering process of clear retainers. Once the system is in place, people will be able to get the retainers they need in a timely fashion and your office won't have to spend a lot of time in the process. You can quickly give patients what they need.

Owning the area of transportation, when it comes to something like clear retainer delivery, means there will be a driving force that patients them moving along. There won't be backups and delays. The flow is maintained so that people get what they need in a timely manner, with very little effort from your office staff. With our tracking and automation system, patients can be impressed or scanned for a clear retainer in one office location and pick up the appliance at a different location. There's no guesswork on where the retainer is located, who fabricated it or when and where it will be delivered. We track every step of the process in our automated software.

Referral Network

The importance of having an excellent referral network cannot be understated. It can literally make or break your practice. A great referral network will provide you with a steady supply of new patients. A poor referral network will leave you cursing your practice and wondering what is missing (it's the excellent referral network that is missing, trust me). I know all too well just how imperative a great referral network is to an orthodontic practice.

Owning the area of transportation means that you will have mastered the art of maintaining and nurturing a wide and diverse referral network. Doing so will provide a stead flow of new patients. Life is a bit like a river. If you keep the water flowing, the river flourishes, remains fresh, and thrives. If for some reason the water is slowed down or stands still, things become stagnant and there's no progress or growth. This is essentially the idea behind owning the area of transportation. It keeps things moving, fresh and encourages growth.

Having spent time with many orthodontists around the world, I know for a fact that most do not have a great referral system in place. That is at least until they work with me and I help them to realize the importance of it and help them achieve the fundamentals of getting one in place. Once you realize how important it is and how to put it into action and maintain it, you will see the kind of growth you desire. Once you see just what it can do for your practice, you will quite honestly wonder why you didn't own this area years ago.

You probably realize the importance of establishing and maintaining a great referral network but you don't know where to start. Perhaps you had a great referral network years ago and you let it get stagnant. Fair enough.

When properly implemented, a strong referral network sends new patients to your office from a wide variety of referral sources, rather than putting all of your eggs in one basket and only getting referrals from just a couple of general dentists or pediatric dentists.

The idea of having a network for your referrals means that there's more to it than just hoping the dentist down the road sends people your way. A great referral network reaches out to all sorts of possible referring sources, such as dentists, hygienists, hospitals, school nurses, pediatricians, ear nose and throat specialists and anyone else who may at some point have the need to refer a patient to an orthodontist.

A great referral network means that you know exactly where each of your new patients comes from and you spend the appropriate amount of time, with boots on ground, visiting and nurturing those referral sources. Far too often, actually most of the time, doctors don't take the time to find out how a new patient ended up going to their office. Without that knowledge, there is no way to know what is working, what isn't, and where you should focus your efforts more and where to back off in other areas. The most successful orthodontists accurately track the source of every new patient.

A great referral system not only tracks where every referral comes from, but it also identifies your referral VIPs. When you have that information you can use it to help increase your referrals. You must make your best referral sources feel extra special. The best way to do that is to build a relationship with them and send them reminders that you appreciate every referral they send your way. Designate a team member or two who will take time to visit with your referral sources. Automate their quarterly schedule in your CRM software. Invite each referring professional to a continuing education event at least twice per year. If you're not visiting personally with each referral source twice per year, someone else is and they are going to steal that referral source from you.

Great referral networks also focus on identifying those top current or former patients who send you high quality referrals. Notice I said "high quality" sources, because not all of them will qualify as being such. There are some referrals that are going to be better than others. Those are the people who are ready to begin treatment, they are easy patients to work with and they are the kind of patient who makes you wish you had at least a dozen more just like them. The best way to get a dozen more just like them is to identify the source that sent them to you and then focus on the relationship with that person.

When you get a referral, do you immediately send a handwritten thank you note to the person or office that sent it your way? Do you have a few VIP events throughout the year for your top referral sources, where you treat them to some great food, entertainment and prizes? How often do you stop by to visit your top referral sources at their offices?

If you are like most other orthodontists, these are things you are either not doing at all or you are doing haphazardly. Either way, it's not paying off or helping you to get more referrals. That's where having a great referral network comes into play, because when you own the area of transportation you will have a system for visiting and reaching out to these centers of influence consistently throughout the year.

Owning It

Imagine your office having multiple locations, an efficient clear retainer delivery system and an amazing referral network. What would that do for your bottom line? Would that help you to get further down the path toward your goals? My guess is that owning this area, the area of transportation, would give you the opportunity to far exceed the dreams and goals you might have for your practice.

One of the best ways to extend your reach, by being able to serve more patients where they are, is to have multiple locations. Not only will you expand your reach with being able to offer convenience to patients, but you will also be able to build more relationships with nearby dental offices, which will become an important part of your referral network. Being able to expedite clear retainer delivery, see more patients by expanding the area you service, and by having an efficient referral network, you will take your practice to a new level.

Remember, you don't have to do every one of the areas in this book, but you must pick one, own it and do it better than it's ever been done before.

"When the customer comes first, the customer will last." - Robert Half

---

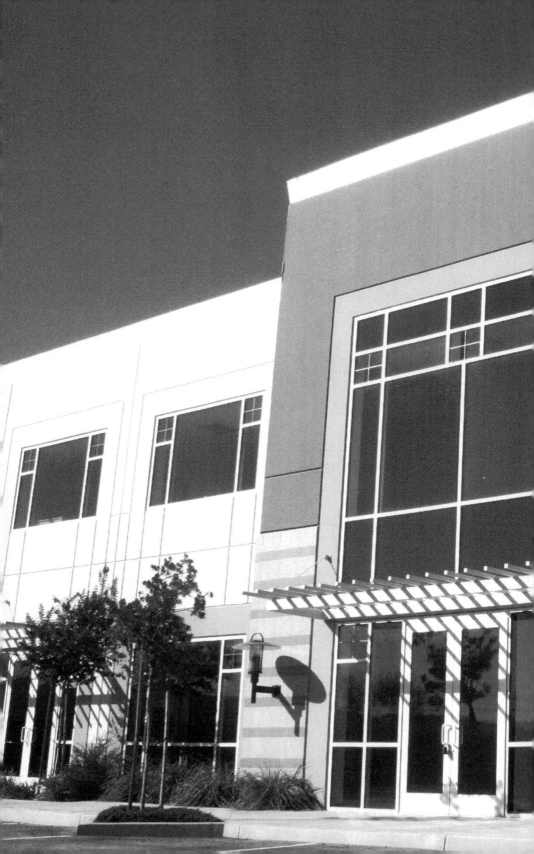

CHAPTER FIFTEEN
REAL ESTATE

"Management is doing things right; leadership is doing the right thing." – Peter Drucker

The great thing about choosing one area to own and doing it better than anyone else is that you have plenty of options. This book has provided you with many options and ideas to consider, and you may even be able to identify some beyond what you read about here. *Owning an area and doing it better than anyone else will set your practice apart and help you thrive.* Believe it or not, it's not so important which area you choose to own, it just matters that you own it completely.

Real estate is another area that an orthodontist will want to consider owning. It's one that can go a long way toward helping your practice become a huge success. I know what you are thinking. Real estate is probably the last thing that orthodontists have on their mind. You would probably be correct, because it's something that most people don't consider, unless an issue comes up that forces them to think about it. Hopefully, this chapter will get you thinking about it long before it's become an issue that you have to take on without prior warning or thought.

With real estate, there are several things that I consider to be important. I have learned about these things through trial and error in my own practices, as well as having gained tremendously valuable insight after watching thousands of hours of secret shopper video, and by providing consulting services to orthodontists around the world. These opportunities have given me a unique perspective that helps identify what is missing, what needs to be done and what can help a practice go straight to the top.

143

Of course, these are not the only options out there. Without a doubt, you will have some of your own that you have identified or that come to mind once you read this book and it helps to get the creative juices flowing.

Facilities Management

Hopefully, you have a busy office. A busy office means that you provide a high volume of treatment and maintain a steady flow of new patients. Of course, it could also mean that your office is disorganized and that your staff is not effective at scheduling patients. I've seen both scenarios, so I realize both ways are possible. The important aspect that I want to refer to here with facilities management is that you are busy, yet also productive.

The physical management of your office and maintenance of the building can be demanding. First of all, it's important to have your building and office in world-class condition. Patients will notice immediately if there are maintenance issues or if things are in disrepair. Patients and parents pay attention to heating and cooling that doesn't work properly, offices and buildings in need of a fresh coat of paint and carpeting that needs a professional steam cleaning. They notice more than you think they do.

The things patients notice about your office make a statement about your attention to detail. If you walked into an office building and it looked shabby or things were falling apart, you would notice right away. You would also form an opinion about the office because of what you see. You can't help but do it, even if you feel you wouldn't hold it against them. Old and outdated faucets, broken ceiling or floor tiles and other cosmetic and functional issues can go a long way toward helping people form opinions about your practcie.

There's a fine line you have to draw between spending time to ensure your building is well maintained and in making sure that your time is spent caring for your patients. You want and need to do both of these things if you want to be highly successful. The more time you spend caring for facility management, the more you are taken away from other tasks. In order to provide you with a better return on your investment, delegate this area of facilities management to a competent employee or third-party vendor with your oversight.

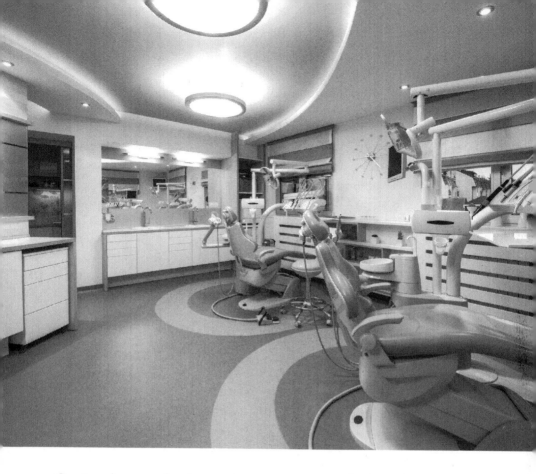

Owning the area of real estate is a great way to meet the tasks at hand and keep your building looking top-notch. You know the importance of having real estate that looks great, functions properly and is well received by your patients. It will help with your professional image, your reputation and in keeping patients happy. When you have happy patients, you not only have people who keep returning for treatment, but there's a good chance that they will refer others to your office as well.

It's imperative that your facility be in the best shape. It must be clean, well maintained, and be a place where patients feel comfortable. In order to own the area of facilities management, it's important that contractors are all in order, their maintenance schedules are automated, that everyone knows who to call and how to handle issues and that you have a process in place with appropriate oversight. If you rent, then this includes managing your lease.

When it comes to your lease, there are things you should know, including what you are allowed to do with the building, if and when there will be rent increases and whether or not you have the ability to sublet a portion of your space to a pediatric dentist or other dental specialist.

Keeping up on each of these areas can be simplified and automated, if you decide to own the area of real estate. If you do, you will find that automating it and simplifying it will keep your facility in top shape, and yet you will no longer be running around trying to get things done all on your own. You don't have to be the person who manages this. Someone in your office can probably own it and do it better than you. It's important to identify the right person for the job and then oversee it by having the person report to you on a consistent, agreed-upon schedule. Putting someone in charge of this who understands the importance of facility maintenance will go a long way toward insuring your practice looks great, functions smoothly and that your patients like what they see.

Far too often, orthodontists get bogged down with the minor details of managing their office buildings. I've heard plenty of horror stories about how leases came up for renewal and the new rate was through the roof. Taking care of these issues and coming out on top is a great thing for your practice. Your building will look beautiful, work efficiently and you will either have the benefit of owning your own building or be able to negotiate a lease that is comfortable and mutually beneficial when you own this area.

It's also important to consider the benefits of owning the building, rather than leasing. There are many advantages to owning your building, including having more control over the layout and changes made to it, your monthly investment is stable, you will have the authority to sublet, should you want to bring in a pediatric dentist and you might realize several tax advantages. Plus, rather than pay into a never-ending lease, you will grow your net worth and enhance your investment income when you are ready to retire.

Owning the buildings for your practices might be a good business move and an investment that will bring about numerous benefits along the way. Depending on the vision you have for your practice and your exit strategy, you should give serious consideration to going this route. In many markets and in certain desirable locations, it might be difficult to purchase your own building, but that doesn't excuse you from managing and maintaining it properly, even if your landlord doesn't take this as seriously as you do.

Population Trends

Keeping up with population trends can have a major impact on your practice. Not keeping up with them can do the same, only in a negative way. When it comes to this issue, you are either keeping up with the trend, watching it pass you by or completely missing the boat. There are many different trends that can have an impact on your practice and keeping up with them makes good sense. It keeps you in touch with your target market and helps you determine the best ways to reach new patients.

Knowing some things about population trends can go a long way toward helping you build and maintain relationships with your target market. For example, the younger population has embraced technology and social media. This means you can reach them on in-app advertising and social media platforms easier than you might be able to reach them through traditional methods. Millennials are a group that as a whole tend to choose experiences over things. This is something that can help you in marketing to them, because giving them straight teeth and a beautiful smile is just the beginning. They expect you to straighten your teeth. How will you make it an experience they cherish and share with their friends and family?

You can use all of the information regarding trends to your advantage. Whether it's trends in bullying, teens wanting Invisalign, or parents seeking Saturday hours for their kids' appointments because they have sports during the weekday evenings, there are plenty of trends to learn. Knowing that bullying is a problem in your area, you can use that angle to help market to your target market. Explain the benefits of straight teeth and how it helps reduce bullying, especially for those who may have severely misaligned teeth.

Owning this area means that you keep up on the trends with your prospective patients, dentists, referral sources, and the industry. Then you use it to benefit both you and your target market. Remember, when others benefit from something you are doing or offering, you will benefit as well. Doing good for them will also produce good returns for you.

There are numerous ways you can go about keeping up with trends, and you don't necessarily have to do them all. Just pick some of them to start out with, so you can gain some useful knowledge. You can do this by checking out trade journals, consumer magazines that your target market would read, taking a look at discussion boards where your target market may frequent, through networking, attending conferences and events and by taking a look at what your competitors are doing.

You can also gain a lot of information about trends just by keeping your eyes and ears open to your own current patients. You would be surprised how much you can learn about them and others like them by paying attention. Notice what they wear, how they talk, what they care about and what they are planning to do. Ask them questions so you can see what their responses may be and if it gives you further clues about who they are and what type of trends are big at the moment. You can even ask them what they think the latest trends are.

When you understand consumer trends, you can use them to your advantage in order to welcome more new patients and build stronger relationships with your existing patients. Referrals are built on the foundation of strong relationships. The more you understand the trends impacting your target market, the better your relationships are going to be. That's a good thing for everyone involved.

The teens you want to reach and their parents are all impacted by consumer trends. Your current geographic advantage can be a disadvantage in a decade. Your current competition will not be the same in the future. Getting to know these consumer trends will put you at an extreme advantage. Patients, parents and your referring doctors will appreciate that you have a sense of what is going on with them and their communities. Constantly gather trend data, keep it in your pocket and use it to build a stronger practice.

Owning the area of real estate and facilities management means you will make it your mission to always keep up on trends in your community. Learn how to best use that information so that it benefits you and your patients.

Practice Consolidation

Another area of real estate to consider is consolidation. Doing this can make a huge difference in your practice. Our practice has done this and it's been highly successful. It's a great way to bring in a steady supply of your own referrals. Rather than relying upon other dentists in your area to send referrals your way, you acquire your own referral sources, like pediatric dental practices, yourself.

At our orthodontist office, we brought in pediatric dentists. Consolidating orthodontic and pediatric dental practices streamlines the referral process. Those patients who start out seeing the pediatric dentist will continue with us if they need orthodontic treatment. There's no need to send them anywhere else. Those patients who come directly to our orthodontic practice might like we have a pediatric dentist in the office and make the switch to seeing that provider. It brings in patients for both, so everyone benefits.

The patient benefits from practice consolidation as well. No longer do they have to go to several offices, deal with additional billing or keep track of separate appointments. People love that their child can come to our office for their teeth cleanings and check-ups, as well as for orthodontic treatment. It brings a higher level of trust, comfort and convenience that is hard to beat. Parents can save time by coming to one location.

In addition to these, there are numerous other benefits to practice consolidation, including:

- **Being able to reduce your costs.** By having another practice or dentist come into your office, they will help share the burden of overhead and facilities maintenance. This helps keep your costs down, even if you want to build a bigger, nicer location.

- **Increased revenue opportunities** are a major benefit to opting for practice consolidation. Your office will have an increase in the number of patients as a result of the consolidation, which will lead to an increase in your annual revenue.

- **Public and professional image.** When your office expands to offer pediatric dentistry, that sends an image to the public. The appearance is one of increased success and authority in the field. People will like the fact that you offer both and see it as a sign of prestige and success.

- **Streamline patient services.** Having a consolidated practice will help to streamline all of the interaction with patients. They will have one contact point, rather than juggling appointments at multiple offices.

Most dentists work solo, which means that they absorb all of the fees and overhead that is involved in doing so. They take on a big risk and they may or may not be happy with the return. When you bring doctors into your office and consolidate practices, you will also be doing them a favor. Their overhead and costs will dramatically decrease, they will gain from your experienced staff backing them up and they will have the ability to gain some of your patients as new ones for themselves.

When it comes to practice consolidation, you have to determine what makes sense for your area. In most cases, bringing in a pediatric dentist is going to make perfect sense. Parents appreciate having a great pediatric dentist available to them, and having that person work right out of your office is just the icing on the cake. It's a situation that will benefit everyone involved.

There are obvious downsides to practice consolidation. With increased size comes increased complexity. To mitigate these risks, consolidate with the right person, at the right time and in the right location. It's also wise to have all of the details written out so that both parties know what is at stake and what the expectations are. The most important part of any contract is the "pre-nup" that explains exactly how the arrangement is going to be unwound, in the event things don't work out. I can't tell you how many times this has saved my rear end and lots of stomach lining.

Don't jump at the first person who is interested in consolidating. You have to find a good match for your office. If you bring in someone with the personality of wet paint, you harm your practice. Always take the person into consideration, as well as the services that will be offered. The person you bring in needs to have the type of work ethic that is shared by your office or that complements it in a nice way. Ask yourself if the person you're about to bring under your roof could have done the same things you have done over the years in building your practice. If the answer is no, keep looking.

As practice overhead continues to rise, it just makes sense to consider practice consolidation. With the right person or group, there are many benefits and very few reasons not to do it. Offering pediatric dentistry through consolidation and acquisition in our orthodontic offices has been a tremendous asset.

Owning It

Owning the area of real estate brings with it a wealth of opportunity. Remember, you don't have to pick all of the ideas presented in this book, but you do have to pick one, and then own it. Do it better than it's been done in your area. When you do that, you will stand out, rise above, and your practice will climb the ladder of success higher than others around you. The vast majority of orthodontic offices never pick something to own, and in doing that they fall short and never reach the level of success that they would like or that they otherwise could.

When you own the area of real estate, you will put your efforts into focusing on facilities management, population trends and in practice consolidation. Don't let this seem overwhelming to you, because when you break down each area and make the decision to go forward, it won't be. There's a good chance that once you get it all in place you will wonder how you ever managed without it. The area of real estate is a major area that is critical to becoming highly successful.

You may find additional areas that fall into the real estate category, too. But the three presented here are tried and true ones that I have learned a great deal about through my own personal experience, by watching all those secret shopper videos and by consulting other orthodontists around the world. Take my word for it when I say that owning this area can take you many places, with all of them pointing up.

"You never get a second chance to make a first impression." - Will Rogers

---

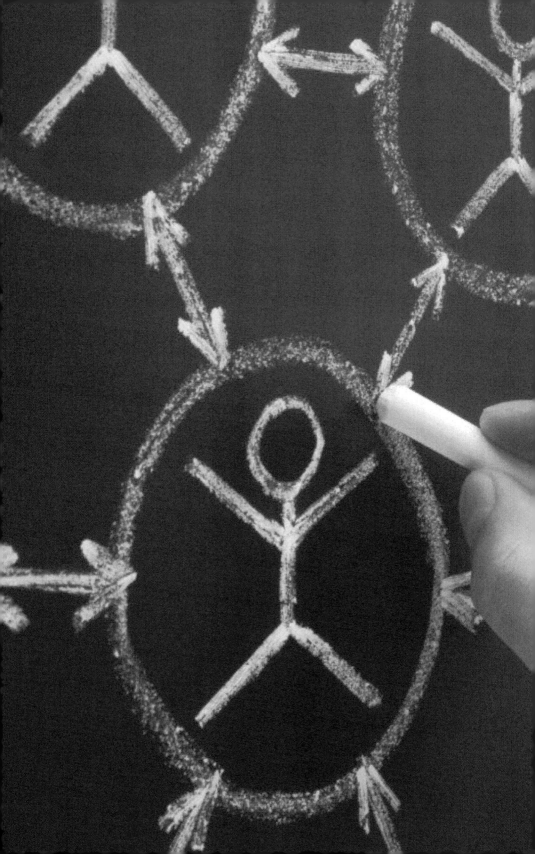

CHAPTER SIXTEEN
PHILANTHROPY

"Think of giving not only as a duty but as a privilege." – John D. Rockefeller

Most people want to do something to help make the world a better place. They might not know how to go about doing so, but their heart is usually in the right place. As an orthodontist, you are in a position where you can do something to help others in your community and you can make a real difference. The philanthropy that you do in your community can be exactly what sets you apart from the competition and puts you ahead of the game.

Of course, nobody goes into philanthropy to gain and become successful from having done so. Let's just get that out there from the start, so that people don't have a warped sense of why owning the area of philanthropy would even be suggested. You don't help others expecting that it's going to help you. That's not how it should work and thankfully, for the majority of people who believe in pursuing philanthropic avenues, they understand this principle.

There often comes a time in one's life when they feel there is something bigger than themselves, or that there is a higher sense of purpose in their life. They might have difficulty determining exactly what that higher sense of purpose is, but if they take the time to explore it and figure it out, the end result can be quite fulfilling.

Higher Purpose

In the field of psychology, this can be explained using Maslow's hierarchy of needs. His theory, which is a pyramid of the needs of each person, starts at the bottom and works its way up to the top of the pyramid. Working your way up the ladder, you have already met your basic needs, as well as your psychological needs for the most part. Some may still be at the point of needing to fulfill the esteem needs of finding prestige and having some sense of accomplishment. But once you have done that, and many of you already have, the next and highest level on the hierarchy is that of self-actualization.

This occurs when you have reached your full potential and you turn your attention to helping others. This is where philanthropy comes into play. When you turn your attention toward helping others, you are going to make a difference in the world around you. As an orthodontist, you have the ability to get involved in one or more causes and make your community a better place.

What happens when you make your community a better place because you have embraced philanthropy? People will take notice. They will see that you care about your community, and that you believe in something bigger than yourself. Only good things can come from this, including the respect that you will get from those in your community. You will also experience wonderful peace in your life.

Creating Smiles

Philanthropy is something I have taken part in for years. I believe in the mission of helping people, and I feel grateful that I've been able to use my skills to help others have a better quality of life. I came from a family of dentists. There are 12 of them in my family, so taking care of teeth and helping others smile with confidence is a bit engrained in me.

At the heart of the charity work that I do is helping those who are born with cleft lip and cleft palate. Serving as the director of the Leo H. Rheam Foundation for Cleft and Craniofacial Orthodontics, I am able to help a cause that is greater than myself. I am also a supporter of the charity Smiles Change Lives. My mission, my higher cause, is to share my time and talents, helping every deserving child enjoy the benefits of a healthy, confident smile.

We've embraced this as our mission in our practices and we've committed to

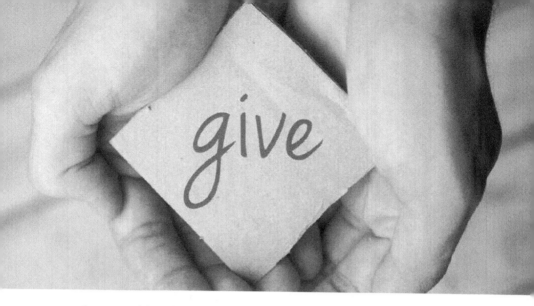

providing over $1 million in free orthodontic treatment each year. That's not a typo. Most orthodontists treat one or two pro-bono cases per year. In the year of this writing, my clinics treated 272 orthodontic cases for free. A goal that big is only possible if your entire team embraces a higher sense of purpose. That's exactly what we've done.

We all know the power of a confident smile. It opens doors and gives one the confidence they need to make a positive difference in their life and in the lives of others. With your skills, you can give more people this gift. Why would you hold back? Not everyone can afford orthodontic treatment. No matter how many payment plans you can come up with, there will always be some people in situations who cannot afford to get the work done to fix their teeth, and without charitable assistance they will likely be left behind. Working with Smiles Change Lives is a great way to make this happen.

This is not to say that the only philanthropic work that you embrace has to be related to someone's smile. If there is a cause that is near and dear to your heart, you should pursue and support it. Another option is to support both, the one you feel passionate about that isn't related to teeth, and also support one that is related to helping people love their smile.

By owning the area of philanthropy, you will stand out as a leader in your community. When that happens, not only will you will feel great, but good things will come back to you. Smiles Change Lives patients aren't poor, they are low income. Their parents work hard and need a hand up, not a hand out. They invest in the program and they will send referrals your way. They have become a massive marketing department for my practice. Many become cash-paying patients when they get back on their feet. Your practice will receive great publicity and you will build a vision of abundance and generosity within your employees.

Others Do it, Too

This is not a new concept, the idea of becoming a philanthropist. The most successful people the world are involved in charitable work. No matter what they have done to become highly successful and earn their living, philanthropy is one thing they all seem to have in common. Most of them give back to those in need by helping a charity or cause that means something to them.

Here is just a sample of some highly successful business people who are giving back through philanthropy:

- **Michael Dell** – The computer giant has given $1 billion to various charitable causes. His area of interest lies in education, health, and in helping families. He also gave a lot to help support growth in the Austin, Texas area.

- **Warren Buffett** – The amount of money that this man has given to help charitable causes is one that would be difficult for anyone else to ever match. In just one year, he gave $26 billion to charity, and he's pledged to give the bulk of his estate, 99% of it, to charity once he passes on. With that kind of funding, he can and does support a wide variety of causes, including health, education, children and community services, and economic development efforts.

- **Tony Hawk** – The professional skateboarder wanted to see kids around the country have a chance at taking up the sport. So, he gave $5.5 million in funding to 572 skateparks, giving kids a place to go skate. It's estimated that 5.5 million people visit the skateparks that he helped fund each year.

Those who are highly successful usually give back to a cause bigger than themselves. They may give to a variety of charities and causes, as Buffett does, or they may have one that they are passionate about, such Tony Hawk, but they tend to give and they give big. One thing Buffett has explained before is that some people can give their time and some can give money. He gives money, because he doesn't have the time to dedicate to charity. By donating money, he helps support the mission and others who have the time to give.

The amount you give is your decision but I encourage you to think big. Disney gave $400 million to charities in 2016. While they are at one end of the spectrum, there are others at the other end, and millions who fall somewhere in between. Again, there's no right or wrong answer here. You want to give enough to make a difference and make it a stretch goal. Don't compare your giving to others but compare yourself to where you were last year. Are you giving more? Are you doing more to help others this year than last year? Commit to doing more and more each year. It will change your life.

We all want the world to be a better place. What can be better than starting by making your own community a better place? If everyone did something to help improve their own community, we would see amazing things happen around the nation and world. Owning the area of philanthropy, you will be in a prime position to help make the community a better place and know that you are doing your part and then some.

Donating Time or Money

With this chapter and idea of owning philanthropy, I can imagine that some of you are left scratching your head, wondering how you would ever fit this in. I get it: We all have very busy schedules and it's difficult to see how you can fit in something else on top of it all. If we only had room for all of the things that would just take "one more hour," it would be great. But since our hours each day are limited, we have to fit in what we can.

You absolutely should be picky about where your time is spent. You only have so much of it and you need to get the most out of it. Your time needs to be spent cultivating relationships with your family, friends and patients. You need to put time into the office, providing treatment and ensuring your office is running like a well oiled machined. You also need to time to relax, read and re-boot. So where does that leave your contribution to charity? Well, that's up to you.

In owning the area of philanthropy, you have two choices. You can choose one or the other, or a combination of both. You can donate some of your time, or you can donate some of your money, or you can do a combination of both. Personally, I tend to both. I donate some of my time to the mission of helping people get the treatment they need that they may not otherwise be able to afford, but also support charities that help those causes I believe in strongly.

You decide how many hours per month or year that you will help with local charities, or how much money you will donate. The choice is completely up to you and there's no right or wrong answer here, it's a matter of what works for you and your family. But the bottom line is that you must focus on something bigger than yourself and have a higher sense of purpose. As orthodontists, we have tremendous potential to change so many lives. How are you living up to your God-given potential? It's up to you to determine how much you want to do, but I encourage you to make it a big goal.

If you decide that making a financial contribution is the best way to go about supporting charity, then great. But there's one thing that I like to share with people about this route that I hope you will take into serious consideration. Let's say you decide that you will start out donating $100,000 per year to help make your community a better place. You find a list of charities you want to support, and you dole out the money, piece by piece, writing little checks to each of the charities on your list. They get the check, they are grateful and all is well.

If we are honest with ourselves, we know that the amount we gave them isn't going to do much. Whether it was $500 or $1,500, there's not a whole lot that most organizations can do to further their mission with small donations. It takes a lot of donations like that to add up to enough to be able to support their efforts. Fingers crossed, they get 10 more donations just like it this year, but that's still a drop in a bucket.

But what if you took your $100,000 donation and you gave it to one or two charities? Choosing those that mean the most to you and your mission, or that you feel will have a major impact in your community. Could a charity do something with a $50,000 or $100,000 donation? Without a doubt, a donation that size will go a long way toward helping further their mission and vision. It will make a real difference in your community.

You make a big statement and you get a lot of results if you make that donation to one, or maybe two charities, rather than trying to dole it out to a long list of organizations. When you do that, you water down the effectiveness. If you want to make real change, give it to one place you believe in and see what it does for that organization. By supporting that one charity with sizeable donations, you will be providing effective help and you will be noticed for that.

One other thing that is important to note when speaking of donating to charities is legitimacy. There are some charities out there that are not good and that do absolutely nothing. You want to make efforts to steer clear of such charities, focusing on only those with a good reputation. It's important to make sure that your donation goes to a charity that is doing what it says it is doing. Investigate the charity before you decide to give it the money, so you can feel comfortable that it will do the right thing.

I recommend CharityWatch.org if you want to see how much of your donation will be used directly in serving the intended recipients of each charity. You would be shocked to discover how many well-respected and famous non-profits use 90% of their donations for administrative costs. One popular charity pays its board members up to $400,000 each per year. You might guess that I don't send them a penny. I prefer organizations that use the lion's share of my donations directly in serving the patient.

You have numerous options when it comes to owning philanthropy, including starting your own foundation, giving your time and donating money to help support many charities. I mentioned that the majority of highly successful people give to help others, but what you might not realize is that many do so through their own charitable foundation. Often times, they create a charity of their choice, that serves their own mission and higher purpose. There are benefits in starting your own charity, including that it's a rewarding experience to have your own foundation. When you do so, you can take an issue that you feel passionate about, such as helping low income children to get free orthodontic work for example, and helping to further that mission to make a real difference.

Additionally, when you start your own charity, as opposed to giving to someone else's, you will leave a legacy for the impact that you make. Although you will have a board, you will also have more say over where the money goes and what types of programs and issues you will focus on. Having more control, leaving a legacy, and finding it personally rewarding are all benefits. I started my own non-profit in order to streamline the process and see results faster. I disliked waiting for cleft kids to get approved for Medicaid or other forms of public assistance, so I simply started doing them on my own. I didn't have to wait and the kids got the right treatment at the right time.

Your practice can benefit in numerous ways by owning the area of philanthropy. Your team morale will go up. They will appreciate that their efforts are making the world a better place. You will also have a great company image that appeals to professionals and generates more referrals.

Benefiting from Philanthropy

As mentioned, you shouldn't go into philanthropy to try to get something in return, or to capitalize on the efforts. That should never be your mission, because the whole idea of philanthropy is to give to others, lift others and help better your community and humanity.

Having said that, and I do hope that point hits home, it is important to know that you can still get a lot of benefits from owning the area of philanthropy. You must know that, or there's not an orthodontist out there who would pick this element to own. After all, this book is about the importance of picking one area, owning it, and doing it better than it's ever been done in your market. That way, you stand out, rise above and take your practice to the highest level that you can.

Fast food giant Dave Thomas, of Wendy's fame, once said that "The more you give to others, the more you get in return." Having been adopted as a child, his philanthropic passion was helping children to find forever homes. There's no doubt about the fact that he gave to this belief not to get something other than feeling that he was making a difference in a cause he believed in. Still, you can't help but to think nice thoughts about the late Thomas, no matter what your feelings are about Wendy's, because his heart was in the right place and he made a difference in the world.

Everyone who owns the area of philanthropy gains benefits like this. It leaves a legacy and creates an image of you that people appreciate. More people are likely to think favorably of you and respect you for the efforts you put forth to help make improve and support the community. Giving back always comes back to you, even if that's not why you gave in the first place.

In order to gain anything from your philanthropy work, whether it be more referrals, respect or to leave a legacy, people need to know about it. This is where your marketing and public relations skills will come into play. Whatever route you take in your philanthropic decisions, be sure to let the community know about them. People should know how and when you are helping others.

You can do this in a variety of ways, such as putting it on your website, sending out press releases, creating videos, posting to social media platforms and so on. Use your marketing efforts to put it out there and let everyone know that you believe in giving back and helping your community. People will always appreciate that you do that, and it may be the deciding factor that motivates people to go to your office for treatment, as opposed to someone else.

Owning It

Philanthropy is just one area out of many that you can choose to own. I've seen practices own it and do some amazing things with it. If you have a passion for helping others and want to help make your community a better place, then this may just be the area that you want to choose to own. If you feel you want to grow your sense of higher purpose, this area is the one for you.

There's a good chance that you will never regret getting involved in philanthropy. There's a widely held belief that when you give to others you get back in return. Not only do you get a great feeling from helping other people, but you are rewarded for your kindness. It's difficult to beat an element that is going to leave you feeling great and mean good things for your practice, while also helping to change the lives of others. Everyone wants a better world, but not everyone wants to put in the effort to help make it happen. Real change starts with each and every person, and by owning the area of philanthropy you will take the bull by the horns and make great strides as you do so.

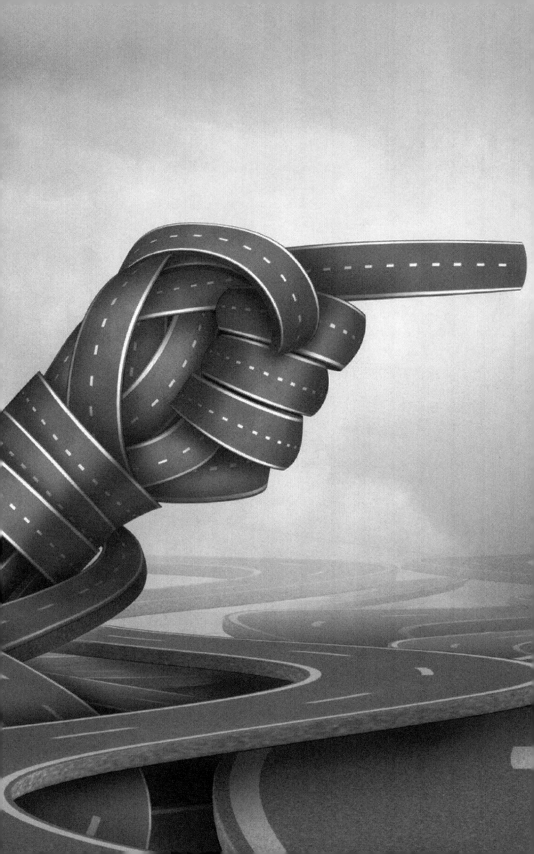

CHAPTER SEVENTEEN
CLOSING THOUGHTS - LOOKING AHEAD

"In any moment of decision, the best thing you can do is the right thing, the next best thing is the wrong thing, and the worst thing you can do is nothing." – Theodore Roosevelt

You have just spent some time exploring 15 areas where I have seen that orthodontists often fall short. The various elements I have proposed here for you to consider are ones that I have learned from personal experience, after watching thousands of hours of secret shopper videos and through the consulting work that I do with orthodontists around the world.

Every orthodontist in the country, unless there's something seriously amiss, wants to have a highly successful practice. They want to stand out, rise above the competition, love what they do and be the best possible leader they can be. Trying to be everything to everyone and fulfill every area often leaves people coming up short. It's hard to hit all 15 of these elements and be the best at them. Your plate can only hold so much, and when you pile on more and more, something inevitably will fall off.

This book isn't about piling on more and more. It's about simplifying more than anything. It's about picking one of these 15 elements and owning it. It's about truly making it your thing and doing all that it takes so that it works for you and helps your practice go straight to the top. My hope is that you got that after reading through and considering each area that you could own and grow.

Making the Choice

People are often afraid to make decisions, simply because they are afraid they will make the wrong one. Psychologically, what goes into our decision making is a whole soup of elements, including reason, our emotions, what others will think, biases and much more. The good news is that there is no right or wrong decision here. As long as you make one, you will not make the wrong choice. The wrong choice is, as Roosevelt said, to close this book and make no decision at all.

If the status quo continues, then you expect exactly what you have been getting all along. If you are happy with that, then great, but since you chose to read this book there is a good chance that you are not satisfied with the status quo. Like many other orthodontists, you are wondering what else you can do to take things to the next level. You wonder where things are falling short.

You took the first step to address what is missing and what you can do to help your practice grow and become more successful. That was reading this book. The next step is to pick one of the elements presented in this book and make the decision that you will own it. You will take the idea, learn everything you can about it, make a plan, carry it out and you will do it better than anyone else in your area has ever done it before.

When you have the decision made as to which one you will own, you will likely feel excited, and you should be. Seeing it through is going to do some amazing things for your practice. A year from now, you will see the fruit of your labor and you will wonder why you never thought of those things before. The truth of the matter is, our brain tends to filter certain things out. We often see things the way we want them to be, rather than for the way they are. You may think you are doing everything great, but a secret shopper video may show numerous areas where your practice is falling short. I've seen it happen many times. It's difficult to see the error of our own ways, which is why my clients go on to have great success when they fix these areas. When someone else looks at your practice in action from a neutral space, it's easy to see where improvements are needed.

A new perspective can often identify the problems holding you back. By choosing one of these areas to own, you will turn your focus to excelling in that

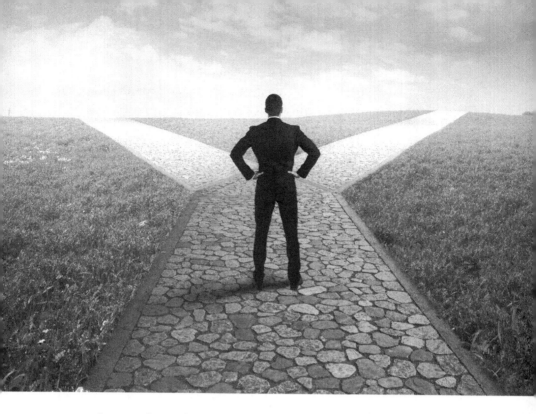

area and you will stand out. When you stand out, you rise above, and when you rise above you will become more successful. You have nothing to lose by giving this a try and everything to gain if you see it through.

While I can offer you these 15 areas to ponder, I can't tell you exactly which one to choose. Only you can do that. I probably don't know you personally, or know your practice and community. This is a decision you will have to make, but it's one that you must make if you want to see big growth in the next 12-18 months.

So how do you go about choosing which area you should own? Here are a few things I recommend you consider to help make that decision:

- **Is there any one particular area that leaped out at you while reading the book?** If there's an area that got you excited or really piqued your curiosity as you read it, then that may be the right one for you. There's a good chance that one of these areas resonated with you more than others, so you may want to start out seriously giving that one some consideration.

- **What are you passionate about?** Are you someone who watches commercials and then picks out the mistakes they make about how they will never reach their target audience with what they produced? Then maybe marketing is the right area for you to focus on. Do you like to work the room, meeting as many people as you can? Then perhaps networking is the right choice for you to make. Do you have a passion for helping others and fulfilling a higher purpose? Then you should explore owning the idea of philanthropy. Every area listed in this book is going to appeal to a different kind of person and personality. Determine which one fits you best.

- **Do you have any particular skill beyond orthodontics that you know you could readily start applying?** For example, in high school and college, I worked in marketing. So right off the bat, I knew that I could hit the ground running with owning the area of marketing. Consider what other types of skills and experience you have, so that you may be able to apply those to picking an area to own. You will be able to step into the role already knowing a great deal, so it will feel comfortable for you.

- **Is there one that stands out because you have a team that works for you that would be able to help pull it off?** If you have a team that works for you that is great at sales, putting on live events, or whatever it is, then that may be your golden ticket. Remember, you don't have to handle every aspect of carrying out the one that you decide to own. The best managers in the world are the ones who know how to delegate and bring out the best in their team, so that objectives and goals are met and the company succeeds.

Reaching the Goal

Once you have decided which element you want to own, it's time to get serious about putting it into action. Most people who set goals, especially ones made around the start of the New Year, never accomplish them. It's not because they don't want the success. They do, but they don't always know how to get there. They don't know what steps to take. We have become accustomed to getting into our car and the GPS gives us a direct plan on how to get from point A to point B. It gives us the fastest route. We have nothing to plan or think about.

When it comes to our goals, we can't just plug our desire into a device and expect it to tell us exactly where to go to avoid pitfalls. We aren't told what challenges will arrive along the way and exactly when we will arrive at our destination. We actually have to do the work. We need to make decisions and plans, carry them out, see them through and follow up. Often we have to navigate around issues and roadblocks when things don't go our way.

To reach any worthwhile goal, you need to do a few things that will help you get there, starting with:

- **Making the commitment.** That's often the hardest step, but the most important. Without it, you will sit idle, without any change or progresss being made.

- **Make a plan.** Once you have made the commitment, make a plan of what it will take to get you to where you want to go. It's taking it old school and pulling out a map so you can come up with route you will take to reach your destination. Break it down into actionable items that you can start doing.

- **Delegate where you can.** There's no way that you can do everything on your own. As mentioned before, the best managers in the world know the importance of delegation and how to bring out the best in their team. Having the right team working on the commitment with you is going to help you reach the top.

- **Revise when and where necessary.** If you started down the road and there was a roadblock, you don't just turn around and go home. Some plans may need to be revised. There's nothing wrong with it, as long as you continue moving toward your goal.

- **Keep your foot on the pedal.** It was Thomas Jefferson who said, "I am a great believer in luck, and I find the harder I work, the more I have of it." Hard work pays off. It's important to be consistent with working toward your goal and in owning it.

- **Stay positive.** It's easy for people to get bogged down if they don't see immediate benefits from their efforts. Don't let that happen. A diamond is not created overnight. Maintain a positive attitude, because what you put out is what you get in return.

- **Hold yourself accountable.** If you don't, you will find yourself slipping and letting yourself get away with it. Coming up with excuses is easy, but they won't lead you to success. Be honest with yourself every step of the way.

As you commit to owning one of these areas, you will see the results begin to take shape. Things will come together and the pay-off will be significant. Each time you see positive results in your favor, you are more likely to press on with a renewed commitment to the goal. Your practice will thrive and you will have an "Own It" mentality that can't be broken. You will see and feel the results of owning it and you will know there's no going back.

Defining What You are Selling

By knowing what it is that you are selling, you will be able to help use that to determine which element you want to own. Many orthodontists are not aware of what it is that they sell. I don't care what you do. Understand what it is that you are selling if you want to be highly successful. Apple's not selling computers and hardware. Uber's not selling transportation. And Domino's is not selling pizza.

These companies defined what they provide very differently. They owned it and they did it better than it's ever been done before. That's what I want for you. That's where I'd see you with our top clients. It's what I see in the secret shopper data. I see 5% of orthodontists out there killing it. They completely own an area and they have risen high above the competition.

If you have ever been to one of our live events, you may have met a few of these clients who are crushing the competition. We have many clients who are consistently converting new patients at 85% and above, some are consistently converting above 90%. Could you imagine what converting 90% of your patients to starting treatment would look like for your practice? What would that do for your future? I've seen what it does for my clients, so I know firsthand how incredible it is for someone's practice when this happens.

The bottom line here is that those practices that have hit the over 85-90% conversion rate defined and owned the idea that they were going to change how they helped people say yes to treatment. They chose it, owned it, and are doing it better than anyone around them. It's quite impressive to see this in action, and I've had the pleasure of seeing it numerous times with the clients I coach.

A lot of people have defined what they want to do. They say something like "We want to be the best orthodontic practice in our area." But the reality is that only the top 1-5% of businesses in any market actually own that position.

It's one thing to say you want to be the best. It's easy to say you want to be the best. That doesn't come with any real commitment to have to actually do something to be the best. It's just lip service unless you actually own it and make it happen.

Owning it means:

- **You stand behind your work.** You provide a satisfaction guarantee. Period. If people aren't happy with you, they get their money back, no questions asked. Sure, you may have just raised your eyebrows at the thought of this, as most orthodontists do. But I've seen what such a guarantee can do. People realize that there's no risk in getting treatment, because if they don't like it then they will get their money back. It's hard not to love such a guarantee. It makes your patients feel comfortable about getting treatment and it shows that you are committed to their happiness. You want them to like the outcome of their treatment, so you are committed to helping them have the best possible experience. That's owning it, and that's hard to beat.

- **You crawl through broken glass for your customers.** It only stings for a little bit. Every one of your patients needs to know that you have their best interest in mind and that come hell or high water, you have their back. You will be there helping them every step of the way, even if it means that once in a while you have to carry them or you admit that you were wrong. When you can provide that level of service, you will own it and you will have the biggest practice in town.

- **You can apologize and admit when you are wrong.** Humans are imperfect. You are going to make mistakes. Don't hide behind a policy or blame someone else. If the patient has decalcification, you can blame the patient, or you can blame your inability to properly motivate them to have the braces taken off a long time ago. Own it. Do whatever it takes to fix it. You will never regret going the extra mile for your patients.

Being Exceptional

I will tell you that I have paid for veneers and composites in too many patients I will tell you that I have paid for veneers and composites in patients with decalcification. Even though we warned them and took out the wires. Even though their dentist agrees that it was the patient's poor hygiene that caused the problem, we still crawl through glass for these patients. And today those patients are raving fans of mine. They send me 10 times more referrals than the cosmetic dentistry costs. Plus, when you have these principles, referring doctors see how committed you are to excellence. You'll be the only orthodontist in your area who behaves like this, and that's exactly what you want.

Anyone can say their business is exceptional. Only the doctors who own it can actually show you the proof.

What happens when you own it? Your revenue and profit will be in the top 1-5% of the profession. Your employee productivity will grow beyond $450,000 in revenue per employee. Referrals will represent the majority of your new patients. New patient conversion will increase to 85% or higher. You will garner a lot of attention in the media. Your fees will tolerate much more elasticity as you're paid for who you are, not what you do.

How does all that sound to you? You may be a little skeptical, but I assure you that those who own it are living this. They are experiencing all of this success and are not looking back or thinking twice. The only difference between them and you is that they made the decision, and they own it. I can't stress that enough to you. *Owning it makes all the difference in the world.*

Success Is Yours

I have every belief in the world that if you apply the principles that I've shared here that you will have amazing success in your practice. Without a doubt I believe that, because I have seen this. Granted, with my consulting clients I work with them one-on-one, so that we can pinpoint what areas in their practice are the ones that need attention. I help them get the ball rolling on what they will own. But I've shared a great deal of insider information with you in the pages of this book, and I hope that it hasn't eluded you.

If you take the information in this book seriously, apply it, get the help where you need it, and remain committed, you will own it and you will soar. I've lived it, seen it, guided others with it, and know that the reward is sweet, sweet success.

You have one person to hold accountable for where your practice is today in terms of success. It's the person in the mirror. And you have only one person to hold accountable for where it will be one year from now and five years from now. That's you.

You hold all the cards when it comes to how successful you want your practice to be. In order to achieve ultimate success, you have to believe that and you have to make the decision to own it.

Once you do that, success is yours and you will find yourself in a small and elite group of orthodontists around the world. We're waiting for you, absolutely want you to succeed and wish you the best of luck in joining us soon.

VISIT **THEBURLESONCHALLENGE.COM**
TO ACCESS THESE FREE RESOURCES:

RECEIVE a free audio disc where Dr. Burleson shares his best internal marketing campaigns and event-based marketing ideas to help you grow your orthodontic practice.

REGISTER for a complimentary on-line training event led by Dr. Burleson, "How to Convert 90% or More of Your New Patients into Starting Treatment Without the Gimmicks or Hype & Without Turning Your Treatment Coordinators into Used Car Salesmen Even if EVERYTHING YOU'VE TRIED Up Until Now Hasn't Worked..."

COMPLETE the Burleson Challenge and see if your practice qualifies to join one of Dustin's private coaching groups where you will work directly with many of the top orthodontists throughout the world and quickly determine the next steps required to take your practice to the next level.

ACCESS ALL OF THE ABOVE FREE RESOURCES BY REGISTERING YOUR BOOK AT
THEBURLESONCHALLENGE.COM